Manual of Sexually Transmitted Infections

This book is dedicated to the memory of my brother,
Kevin Michael Peate.

Manual of Sexually Transmitted Infections

by

IAN PEATE EN(G), RGN, DIPN(LOND), RNT,
BED(HONS), MA(LOND), LLM

Associate Head of School, School of Nursing and Midwifery,
University of Hertfordshire

W
WHURR PUBLISHERS
LONDON AND PHILADELPHIA

© 2005 Whurr Publishers Ltd
First published 2005
by Whurr Publishers Ltd
19b Compton Terrace
London N1 2UN England and
325 Chestnut Street, Philadelphia PA 19106 USA

British Library Cataloguing in Publication Data

A catalogue record for this book
is available from the British Library.

ISBN 1 86156 497 X

Typeset by Adrian McLaughlin, a@microguides.net

Contents

Acknowledgements

I would like to express my specific gratitude to my partner Jussi Lahtinen for all of his continued encouragement and support. I would also like to thank Frances Cohen and Lyn Cochrane.

Introduction

The topics discussed in this text are relevant to all nurses, midwives, specialist community public health nurses and other health care workers, working in the primary, secondary, intermediate and tertiary sectors of health care, the independent sector and the National Health Service. Sexual health matters for everyone; however, sexual health needs vary from one person to another, from one community to another as well as evolving throughout life (Medical Foundation for Sexual Health, 2004).

Some key facts related to sexual health

- There has been an increase across the population related to sexual risk-taking behaviour.
- HIV prevalence in adults has increased by 20 per cent. It is estimated that on average 31 per cent of people who are HIV positive in the UK are unaware of it.
- The most common STI is chlamydia which affects one in ten sexually active young women. If left untreated chlamydia can lead to pelvic inflammatory disease, ectopic pregnancy, infertility, psychological and emotional distress.
- Genital warts have increased by 2 per cent and syphilis by 28 per cent.
- Delays in accessing treatment for STIs can lead to an increase in the number of people infected.

There are inequalities associated with sexual health and the provision of services. Women, young people, gay men, black and ethnic minority groups and people living in London are disproportionately affected (DoH, 2004b). Discrimination is a real threat to persons with STIs; discrimination on the basis of infection (direct or indirect) with an STI is unlawful.

The national perspective

The most influential government report produced to improve the sexual health of the nation was published by the Department of Health in 2001 – the Strategy for Sexual Health and HIV in England (DoH, 2001c). Scotland has a five-tier model of sexual health service provision (Scottish Executive, 2003). The Welsh Assembly has produced their own strategic document (National Assembly for Wales, 2000) and Northern Ireland is currently preparing their own strategy (Department of Health Social Services and Public Safety, 2003). The strategy for sexual health together with the Implementation Action Plan (DoH, 2002d) have been produced to improve sexual health and reduce health inequalities. England is currently experiencing a rapid decline in its sexual health (House of Commons Health Committee, 2003). There is also recognition of the direct links between health inequalities and sexual ill health:

- poverty;
- poor housing;
- unemployment;
- discrimination;
- other forms of social exclusion.

The main aims of the strategy are to:

- reduce the transmission of HIV and STIs;
- reduce unintended pregnancy rates;
- improve health and social care for people living with HIV;
- reduce the stigma associated with HIV and STIs.

Plans are outlined in the strategy that propose a modern, efficient and user-centred sexual health service. There are proposals to abolish the unfair and unjustified variations in access, quality and provision of sexual health services (Medical Foundation for Sexual Health, 2004).

The Sexual Health Strategy (DoH 2001c) states that there should be a new model of working, with three levels of service provision (see Table I.1).

The recommendations made in the Sexual Health Strategy (DoH, 2001c) are to be translated into practice by the provision of Sexual Health Leads at each Primary Care Trust (PCT). For nurses this will have implications: the role of the nurse will be further extended and autonomous practice will be enhanced.

The Royal College of Nursing has produced their own sexual health strategy (RCN, 2001) providing further guidance for nurses. The strategy provides guidance that will help the nurse work more effectively in the field of sexuality and sexual health.

Table I.1 The three levels of sexual health service provision

Level 1
A basic level of sexual health provision, this is likely to be carried out in a GP surgery or walk-in centre; both of these venues will not provide an enhanced or specialist service. Some of the services offered at level 1 may include:

- The provision of emergency contraception
- Hormonal contraception
- Opportunistic screening for STIs
- Treatment for STIs
- Cervical cytology

Level 2
This level provides care that is offered at an enhanced level; it will include all services offered at level 1 and a degree of specialist provision. Services at this level may include:

- Fitting of intrauterine devices/intrauterine systems
- Advanced genitourinary care that may include the treatment of complicated STIs and contact tracing
- HIV counselling, testing and treatment
- Training for nurses and doctors who may wish to undertake family planning or genitourinary courses

Level 3
Specialist provision of sexual health services that provide most of or all of the above; this level will also provide expertise in research, education and training

Source: adapted from Royal College of Nursing, 2004a.

Nurses caring for patients in the primary care sector, i.e. GP surgeries, might find that their work practices may change with the implementation of the new General Medical Services contract, as some surgeries may opt to deliver sexual health services. These changes can provide the practice nurse with new ways of providing a service with a sexual health focus in some PCTs.

A toolkit has been produced to help those in the PCTs and others who work in the field of promoting good sexual health and HIV services (DoH, 2003a). The aim of the toolkit is to help implement the sexual health strategy at a local level. The Royal College of General Practitioners (2003) provide guidelines for the appointment of general practitioners with special interests in the delivery of clinical services associated with sexual health; the guidance details the core activities of a GP surgery considering offering special sexual health services.

The context and association with other national initiatives

The strategies associated with sexual health are planned and implemented in the context of other programmes and strategies produced by the government; they should not therefore be seen as strategies in isolation. The following provides details of some documents, in addition to those discussed above, that have been produced by the government. They will impinge upon and inform the implementation of the sexual health strategy.

The government's teenage pregnancy strategy (Social Exclusion Unit, 1999) is complemented by the national strategy for sexual health. The aim of this strategy is to address teenage pregnancy and consider some of the reasons behind the high rate of unintended pregnancies in the UK and to set out an action plan, including better campaigning and joined-up, coordinated prevention and support services.

The NHS Plan (DoH, 2001d), a vision for providing a better quality service, was produced in 2001. In this proposal the aim was to provide better quality services, designed around the needs of patients and delivered by a sustained programme of investment and reform.

A radical restructuring of the NHS was undertaken in response to Shifting the Balance of Power produced in 2002 (DoH, 2002e). Decentralization of power and resources occurred and this was devolved to PCTs with the aim of providing better delivery of health care to patients.

Choosing Health: Making Healthy Choices was published in 2004 (DoH, 2004b). The focal point of this publication is to ensure that the most marginalized and disadvantaged groups in our society have the opportunity to see faster improvements in their health.

An international perspective

The above discussion is concerned primarily with a local/national approach to enhancing sexual health services. From an international perspective the WHO (2000) consider sexual health problems as syndromes: they identify eight clinical syndromes (see Table I.2).

The Royal College of Nursing (2004c) has developed a competency framework to enhance the delivery of sexual health care in response to:

- a need for a clear pathway for nurses working in the sexual health and reproductive fields;
- the rapid increase in acute STIs;
- the increase in HIV diagnoses;
- the high rates of teenage pregnancy.

The framework recognizes the further extended role the nurse is likely to

Table I.2 Sexual health problems as identified by the WHO

Clinical syndromes that impair sexual functioning (sexual dysfunction):

- Hypoactive sexual desire
- Sexual aversion
- Female sexual arousal dysfunction
- Male erectile dysfunction
- Female orgasm dysfunction
- Male orgasm dysfunction
- Premature ejaculation
- Vaginismus
- Sexual pain syndromes (including dyspareunia and other pain conditions)

Clinical syndromes related to impairment of emotional attachment/love (also known as paraphilias):

- Exhibitionism
- Fetishism
- Frotteurism
- Paedophilia
- Sexual masochism
- Sexual sadism
- Fetish transvestism
- Voyeurism
- Unspecified paraphilia

Clinical syndromes related to compulsive sexual behaviours:

- Compulsive cruising and multiple partners
- Compulsive fixation on an unattainable partner
- Compulsive autoeroticism
- Compulsive love affairs
- Compulsive sexual behaviour in a relationship

Clinical syndromes involving gender identity conflict:

- Childhood gender dysphoria
- Adolescent gender dysphoria
- Adult gender dysphoria
- Intersex syndromes
- Unspecified gender identity syndrome

Clinical syndromes related to violence and victimization:

- Clinical syndromes following being sexually abused as a child/minor (including but not limited to post-traumatic stress disorder)
- Clinical syndromes following being sexually harassed
- Clinical syndromes following being sexually violated or raped
- Clinical phobia focused on sexuality (e.g. homophobia, erotophobia)
- Clinical syndromes related to engaging in threat or acts of violence focused upon sex or sexuality (e.g. raping another person)
- Patterns of unsafe sexual behaviour placing self and/or others at risk for HIV infection or/and other sexually transmitted infections

Table I.2 continued

Clinical syndromes related to reproduction:
- Sterility
- Infertility
- Unwanted pregnancy
- Abortion complications

Clinical syndromes related to sexually transmitted infections:
- Genital ulcer
  - Non-vesicular
  - Vesicular
- Oral ulcer
  - Non-vesicular
  - Vesicular
- Rectal ulcer
  - Non-vesicular
  - Vesicular
- Discharge
  - Urethral
  - Vaginal
  - Rectal
- Lower abdominal pain in women
- Asymptomatic STIs and infestations (including HIV)
- Acquired Immunodeficiency Syndrome (secondary to HIV)

Clinical syndromes related to other conditions:
- Clinical syndromes secondary to disability or infirmity
- Clinical syndromes secondary to physical or mental illness
- Clinical syndromes secondary to medication or other medical and surgical interventions
- Colorectal conditions
- Clinical syndromes secondary to other conditions

Source: WHO, 2000.

develop in the future and the potential nurses have to improve the outcomes for the patient with respect to their sexual health.

The DoH in conjunction with the Royal College of Nursing (2003b) has stated that what is important to the patient is that they are seen by the right person, with the right skills and competence regardless of whether they are a nurse or doctor. In many situations regarding sexual health and STIs the nurse may well have the right level of competence and skills and s/he may well be the right person to be seen by the patient.

One example of the extension of the nurse's role may be with the use of patient group directions. These directions (previously known as group protocols) are written instructions for the supply or the administration of medicines for groups of patients who may be individually identified before presenting for treatment (RCN, 2001). Patients with STIs may be considered in this respect and as such, the nurse may be involved in patient group directions for managing the patient with an STI.

The competency framework focuses on the patient's experience related to sexual and reproductive health services. There are five competencies addressed by the framework, which are seen as specific to sexual and reproductive health. They are:

- clinical assessment;
- clinical examination and specimen collection;
- interpretation and provision of findings;
- provision of treatments and therapies;
- health promotion.

The competencies are ordered in a way that reflects the patient journey through the sexual and reproductive health services; they are also described across three levels of practitioner:

- registered practitioner;
- senior registered practitioner;
- consultant practitioner.

The need for professional education

In order to provide high quality sexual health services nurses must acknowledge the need to enhance their knowledge, skills and attitudes to do this. Lifelong learning is one way in which the nurse can build upon current skills and enhance the care provided to the patient; professional ongoing education is also needed.

Skilled nurses have pivotal roles to play in HIV and STI prevention, raising awareness of sexual health and helping people to get the services and information they need. Better education of health care professionals and building upon the evidence that is available are central to the success of the sexual health strategies of all four countries in the UK. Staff should have access to flexible, multiple professional education in order to deliver successful health promotion activities. One example of a flexible approach is the Royal College of Nursing's sexual health skills distance learning pack (RCN, 2003b). This initiative aims to improve the levels of sexual health knowledge and skills of Registered Nurses in an attempt to help them contribute towards the sexual health needs of society.

Quality education can help the nurse develop his/her interpersonal and communication skills, as well as their clinical and technical abilities (DoH, 2001a). Section 6 of the Sexual Health Strategy (DoH, 2001c) details issues related to the development of professional education and training for health care staff.

The chapters

Chapter 1 concentrates on health promotion. Health promotion plays a major part in helping the population maximize their health, and this is also true with respect to sexual health promotion which is crucial if the incidence of STIs is to be reduced.

Understanding the key concepts associated with health promotion (the theoretical concepts and theories) will enable the nurse to apply the theories and principles to practise in order to provide high quality sexual health promotion. This chapter provides definitions of complex terms, i.e. health, sexual health and sexual health promotion.

The five strategies associated with the Ottawa Charter are provided for the nurse to use in order to provide a framework for successful sexual health care delivery. The chapter suggests that there are three main categories in which health promotion models can be placed:

• behavioural change;
• self-empowerment;
• collective models.

It is noted that all three models and the elements associated with these models are not mutually exclusive; often all three are used together and interchangeably.

Practical advice and guidance are offered to the reader in relation to the preparation of written patient information. The nurse is encouraged to provide quality information, as any information presented to patients can influence each experience they have with health care provision and providers.

In Chapter 2 emphasis is placed on the importance of obtaining a detailed sexual health history. Taking a sexual health history can be carried out as part of general history taking. This is not the exclusive province of the sexual health nurse: all nurses should develop the skill needed to do this with confidence and competence. The outcomes of the sexual health history can also allow people to receive appropriately targeted advice and information on prevention of STIs, HIV or unintended pregnancies within many clinical settings.

There are practical hints and tips that can ease the novice nurse into the taking of a comprehensive sexual health history. Emphasis is placed on the importance of documentation and the nurse's responsibilities related to documentation and record-keeping.

Chapter 3 provides the reader with much detail relating to the management of STIs. Nine STIs have been chosen and discussed in order to care for patients and their partner(s) with STIs. The nurse needs to have an indepth understanding of the range of conditions with which they may come into contact. Understanding the fundamental facts about the various STIs, and how they may be transmitted, can be the first steps towards preventing them.

Each section related to the STIs deals with a particular infection and specifically addresses – the epidemiology, the causative organism, transmission, the incubation period, clinical manifestations, potential complications, diagnosis, management and subsequent care and any special considerations that may need to be noted. In order to detect an STI the nurse needs to employ practices that are commensurate with high quality nursing and this will include obtaining an adequate specimen from the patient in accordance with local policy; failure to obtain an adequate specimen may be detrimental to a patient's care.

Counselling skills and the skills the nurse needs to communicate effectively with patients who have an STI are highlighted in Chapter 4. The nurse is encouraged to beware of his/her limitations associated with the complexities of counselling. Key terms are defined and discussed in an endeavour to define what is meant by counselling and to differentiate between counselling, using counselling skills and using communication skills.

While it is acknowledged that nurses offer support and give advice to patients in many ways in their everyday work, it is also noted that nurses are not counsellors and as such they need to refer patients to the most appropriate health care professional when they have recognized their limits. The issue of pre- and post-test HIV counselling is also addressed in this chapter.

Chapter 5 centres on the complexities associated with partner/contact notification; these terms are discussed in an attempt to ensure that they are used in the correct and most appropriate way when working with patients, contacts and partners. The processes related to partner/contact notification are described; the advantages and disadvantages associated with the various approaches are outlined. This chapter concludes by suggesting that further research is needed in order to determine the true effectiveness of the various approaches used so as to determine best practice with the best evidence available to support such practices.

There are few areas of health care that are untouched by the law and involvement with the legal process may occur during the course of a nurse's career. Chapter 6 considers the legal, ethical and professional issues which nurses need to consider when working with patients. This chapter draws on professional standards, legislation and ethical/moral theory. A brief overview of the legal system is provided.

It is acknowledged that within the legal/ethical framework conflict can and does occur, so an understanding of the legal and ethical burden placed on the nurse may assist him/her in coming to terms with the potential incompatibility. As a registered nurse, midwife or specialist community public health nurse, the reader is reminded that you are personally accountable for your practice. Adherence to the standards laid down by the profession and acting within the realms of the law are required by the nurse when working with patients and their partners with STIs.

The final chapter, Chapter 7, considers those groups of people in society who are deemed vulnerable when the issue of STIs is being considered. Some groups are considered particularly vulnerable, for example, young people, men who have sex with men, some black and minority ethnic groups and those who have been raped or sexually assaulted. These groups are discussed in this chapter; however, it is acknowledged that there are other groups who may also be deemed vulnerable, i.e. those with learning disabilities, prisoners and intravenous drug users.

Each group is considered individually and the discussion includes insights into their specific needs related to the provision of an effective sexual health service. The discussion regarding young people, for example, provides various definitions of the term 'child'.

Sexual abuse can occur in any society. In this chapter it is addressed specifically in relation to young people and there is a section regarding those adults who have been raped or sexually abused. Practical advice concerning the examination and the forensic examination that may take place after the attack is discussed.

Ubiquitous and insidious, STIs are accountable for much morbidity and mortality locally, nationally and internationally; they are also important co-factors in the sexual transmission of HIV. STIs have a direct and indirect economic impact for society; they are a major cause of productive years lost (Edwards et al., 2001).

While this text focuses upon STIs it must be noted that sexual health is central to our health and well-being. Positive sexual heath has long-term implications for our self-esteem, socio-economic status and livelihood. These implications are influenced by policies related to education, welfare and regeneration. The sexual health 'agenda' now takes up a major role with respect to public health and has been identified by the government in several key documents.

Sexual health must be underpinned by a holistic philosophy, positively endorsing human sexuality and accepting sexual activity as normal and life-enhancing. An integrated approach to the contributing factors surrounding STIs should be considered and the range of influencing dynamics at play addressed.

If the rising numbers of STIs are to be tackled then access to services must be improved and a creative and innovative approach is required to promote an open and healthy environment for sex and sexual relations to take place and flourish in, for all members of our society. An integrated service is advocated; for example, one that embraces local communities and educational programmes. The nurse, in a knowledgeable and informed manner, can contribute to these aspirations in a variety of ways with the patient at the centre.

CHAPTER ONE

Sexual health promotion

Introduction

Understanding the key concepts associated with health promotion will enable the nurse to apply these theories and principles in order to provide high-quality sexual health promotion. Health promotion plays a major part in helping the population maximize their health. Each registered nurse, midwife and specialist community public health nurse must ensure that s/he promotes the interests of patients and clients (NMC, 2004a). One of the ways this can occur is by helping patients gain access to information, i.e. health promotion information. The NMC (2004a) state practitioners must:

> Protect and promote the interests and dignity of patients and clients, irrespective of gender, age, race, ability, sexuality, economic status, lifestyle, culture and religious or political beliefs ... Recognize and respect the role of patients and clients as partners in their care and the contribution they can make to it. This involves identifying their preferences regarding care and respecting these within the limits of professional practice, existing legislation, resources and the goals of the therapeutic relationship.

With the NMC quote above still in mind Pellegrino (1981) states:

> Experts have no special prerogatives entitling them to make judgements for the rest of humankind.

The role of the nurse in association with health promotion is to support the patient by attempting to empower and educate them, to protect them from infection; this is coupled with the aim of also preventing the spread of infection. This often places the nurse in the invidious position of being with a patient who feels they are to blame for their own infection and also the infection of others. The nurse must always avoid the idea of there being an 'innocent party' and apportioning blame.

The aim of sexual health promotion described by the DoH (2003b) is to:

Improve the positive sexual health of the general population and to reduce inequalities in sexual health.

There are more specific aims associated with health promotion such as to:

- reduce the number of cases of new and undiagnosed HIV infections;
- reduce the rates of sexually transmitted infections;
- reduce the numbers of unintended pregnancies;
- reduce psychosexual problems;
- facilitate more satisfying, fulfilling and pleasurable relationships.

The WHO (2000) suggests that as the protection of health is a basic human right, then sexual health involves sexual rights which also deserve protection. There are eleven sexual rights that have been declared as universal (see Table 1.1).

Table 1.1 WHO Declaration of Sexual Rights

- The right to sexual freedom
- The right to sexual autonomy, sexual integrity and safety of the sexual body
- The right to sexual privacy
- The right to sexual equality
- The right to sexual pleasure
- The right to emotional sexual expression
- The right to sexually associate freely
- The right to make free and responsible reproductive choices
- The right to sexual information based upon scientific inquiry
- The right to comprehensive sexuality education
- The right to sexual health care

Source: WHO, 2000.

Defining key terms

In order to provide health promotion that is going to be effective, the starting point must be to define various key terms, i.e.

- health;
- sexual health;
- sexual health promotion.

Health

The term health is complex and there are various definitions available

(Forster et al., 1999). Many issues will impinge upon and influence health (Hampson, 2000):

- personal behaviour;
- environment;
- politics;
- social and genetic factors.

A popular definition of health that has not been amended since 1948 is provided by the World Health Organization (1948). They state that it is:

> A state of complete physical, mental and social well-being and not merely the absence of disease or infirmity.

This definition will allow the nurse to consider the person from three distinct perspectives. Health can be viewed as a positive concept encompassing social and personal resources as well as the individual's physical capability. The interrelationship between all three perspectives is demonstrated in Figure 1.1.

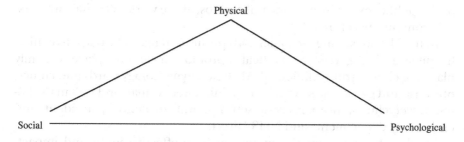

Figure 1.1 The interrelationship of the three key perspectives associated with health. Source: Seedhouse (1986).

Sexual health

While the definition of health per se can be complex, so too can the definition of sexual health as it demands a specific focus. There are, again, many definitions of this term. The WHO (2002a) defines sexual health as:

> a state of physical, emotional, mental and social well being related to sexuality; it is not merely the absence of disease, dysfunction or infirmity. Sexual health requires a positive and respectful approach to sexuality and sexual relationships, as well as the possibility of having pleasurable safe sexual experiences, free of coercion, discrimination and violence. For sexual health to be attained and maintained sexual rights of all persons must be respected, protected and fulfilled.

Sexual health promotion

Any definition of sexual health promotion must include and acknowledge emotional health. In so doing, that definition will make a link between well-being and self-esteem. The following definition of sexual health promotion is provided by the Department of Health (2003b):

> Any activity which proactively and positively supports the sexual and emo-
> tional health and well-being of individuals, groups, communities and the
> wider public and reduced the risks of HIV transmission.

This definition points to the individual, group, communities and the wider population who have the potential to make an active response in taking over control regarding the decisions and choices that will affect their sexual health.

Sexual health promotion may be taken to mean that it takes place in a particular setting, i.e. the practice setting, the GUM clinic or the hospital ward. This is a mistaken belief, as sexual health promotion can and does take place in various settings such as schools, youth centres, residential care settings, institutions of further and higher education, on the streets, in parks, public sex environments, pubs, clubs, at the workplace, hairdressers' and community centres.

In health care settings sexual health promotion may take place in clinics, hospitals and surgeries. Sexual health promotion can take place in family planning clinics, youth clinics, GUM clinics, gynaecology wards and clinics, obstetric and gynaecology wards and clinics, well woman and well man clinics, travel clinics, primary care settings, walk-in centres, accident and emergency departments and NHS Direct.

In all of these venues the nurse can have effective input and impact. However, this does not just involve nurses, midwives and specialist community public health nurses: sexual health promotion activities are delivered by staff from many disciplines in statutory and non-statutory settings, as described above. The nurse must work with others to help promote sexual health of individuals, groups and communities.

Approximately over 90 per cent of patient journeys begin and finish within the primary care domain (DoH, 2002c). Leyshon and Tofts (2004) suggest that this means that the practice nurse will often be the first point of contact for the patient. The practice nurse consults with a wide range of patients of all ages and from all walks of life; because of this it may be suggested that the practice nurse is well placed to promote sexual health.

Sexual health in the general practice

A general practice provides the patient with the opportunity of continuity of care and the provision of a range of services. Some of the objectives of sexual health promotion are outlined in Table 1.2. These objectives and the aims of sexual health promotion can be undertaken with individual patients, specific groups of patients, and the community in general.

Table 1.2 Some objectives of sexual health promotion

Awareness raising

- Increasing awareness of the integral relationship between sexual health and emotional and mental health and enabling the practice nurse to integrate this awareness into his/her practice
- Increasing public awareness of sexual health issues
- Increasing awareness of the importance of positive sexual and emotional relationships

Information and education

- Increasing access to sexual health information, support and advice
- Increasing the levels of sex education and relationships education available to children and young people in particular
- Offering opportunities for adults as well as young people to access sex education and relationships education and to support them regardless of their age or ability

Development of services and service providers

- Increasing access to, and the effective use of, condoms and contraception
- Increasing access to, and uptake of, emergency contraception and abortion services
- Increasing access to, and uptake of, psychosexual and sexual health support services
- Increasing access to HIV and STI testing
- Supporting organizations, service providers and professional staff to play an active role in promoting sexual health

Skills and capacity-building in individuals and communities

- Enabling particularly vulnerable individuals, groups and communities to take greater control over their sexual health
- Offering individuals, groups and communities opportunities to gain key relationship skills such as negotiation, communication, assertiveness, saying no and decision-making
- Enhancing the self-esteem and the emotional and mental health and well-being of individuals, groups and communities

Source: Department of Health, 2003b.

Promoting sexual health

In order to promote sexual health effectively for the various individuals, groups and communities the nurse must engage in a variety of interventions that have to be appropriate and sensitive to the patient's particular needs.

The Medical Foundation for Sexual Health (2004) suggests that the public should have access to:

- consistent, accurate and culturally appropriate information on sexual health (and services);
- effective interventions to minimize risks of STIs and HIV or unwanted pregnancies;
- opportunities to develop the self-efficacy skills to support decisions and choices about sexual health.

The Health Development Agency (HDA, 2004a) has recently undertaken a review of reviews regarding the effectiveness of interventions related to sexual risk behaviours and HIV transmission. They have determined that there is no evidence to suggest that any single intervention can work successfully to reduce risk-taking behaviours – multi-component interventions are recommended. Nurses therefore need to consider health promotion activities from a variety of perspectives. In another review they considered the issue of STIs and the effectiveness of non-clinical interventions (HDA, 2004b). There are many important issues discussed in the report that may help the nurse decide upon the most appropriate approaches to prevention and reduction in risk taking behaviours. This report concludes that more research is needed into what works and (just as important) what does not work, when developing strategies to prevent STIs.

The Ottawa Charter: a framework to promote sexual health

The Ottawa Charter for Health Promotion (WHO, 1986) is a framework that can be used successfully by nurses for sexual health care delivery. The primary aim of the Ottawa Charter for Health Promotion is to attempt to bring about positive long-term changes to the health of communities. The potential role of workplaces, neighbourhoods and schools in improving people's health and reducing health inequalities was highlighted in *Saving Lives: Our Healthier Nation* (DoH, 1999a). *The Health of the Nation* (DoH, 1992) cited cities, schools, workplaces, homes and environments as possible health settings. This approach is derived from the Ottawa Charter which stated: 'Health is created and lived by people within the settings of their everyday life; where they learn, work, play and love.'

Health promotion is defined by the World Health Organization (1986) (The Ottawa Charter) as:

> The process of enabling people to increase control over and to improve their health. To reach a state of complete physical, mental and social well-being, an individual or group must be able to identify and to realize aspirations, to satisfy needs, and to change with the environment. Health is, therefore, seen as a resource for everyday life, not the object of living. Health is a positive concept emphasizing social and personal resources, as well as physical capabilities. Therefore, health promotion is not just the responsibility of the health sector, but goes beyond healthy lifestyles to well-being.

The Charter supports the suggestion that health cannot be understood in isolation from social conditions (Naidoo and Wills, 1998). Hence, wherever people eat, relax and study this has the potential to have a harmful effect on their health.

The strategies within the Charter can help address factors that are within the control of the individual and also those who have their origins in the fabric of society (Cusack et al., 1997). The nurse can translate and use the framework of the Charter to address the sexual health needs of the patient and the community, thereby promoting sexual health.

When considering nursing interventions, nurses need to be aware of the strategies and processes outlined in the Charter. As well as the strategies associated with the Charter there are other skills that the nurse needs to possess or develop in an effort to facilitate the implementation of the Charter (Cusack et al., 1997). These processes – enabling, mediating and advocating – will help to empower the individual and the community to determine their own health promotion activities; they can help place the individual and the community at the centre of any decision-making activities related to their health care needs.

Enabling

Health promotion focuses on achieving equity in health and aims at reducing differences in current health status, ensuring equal opportunities and resources are available to enable all people to achieve their fullest health potential. This will include a secure foundation in an environment that is supportive with access to information, life skills and opportunities in order to make healthy choices.

Mediating

The prerequisites for health cannot be guaranteed by the health sector alone: people from all walks of life contribute at an individual level, through and with families and from various communities. Effective health promotion occurs when there are coordinated activities by governments, by health and other social and economic sectors, by nongovernmental and voluntary organizations, by local authorities, by industry and by the media (WHO, 1986). Nurses and other health professionals have a responsibility to mediate between conflicting interests in society for the quest of health.

Advocating

Health promotion aims at making the political, economic, social, cultural, environmental and biological conditions favourable through advocacy for health.

Health promotion strategies and programmes should be adapted to meet the local needs and possibilities of the individual, taking into account the differing social, cultural and economic systems at play.

There are five strategies (levels) associated with the Charter (see Figure 1.2):

- developing personal skills;
- creating supportive environments;
- strengthening community action;
- building healthy public policy;
- re-orienting services in the interest of health.

There are three stages/levels associated with health promotion: health education, health protection and health prevention. A local sexual health prevention strategy which includes and integrates activities across the range of levels is recommended (Medical Foundation for Sexual Health, 2004). French (1990) suggests that health education is a practical endeavour, focused on improving and understanding the determinants of health and illness and helping people to develop the skills they need to bring about change. Health promotion is a convenient conceptual tool which enables us to order our understanding of those often diverse elements within society that have the potential to promote health.

Building healthy public policy

Policy and legislation are the backbone of the political, legal and social framework for the community and are essential for creating an environment that enables individuals and communities to establish and maintain healthy sexual lifestyles (New South Wales Department of Heath, 2002).

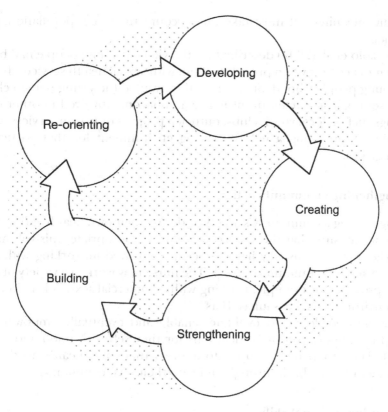

Figure 1.2 The five strategies associated with the Ottawa Charter. Source: WHO, 1986.

The Sexual Health Strategy could be seen as an example of public policy, as is the Healthy Schools Scheme. The Teenage Pregnancy Strategy (Social Exclusion Unit, 1999) is another example of public policy that has an impact on sexual health. Nurses can be involved with the implementation of these policies at a local level and can contribute to local public health policy through health improvement programmes (HImPs). HImPs, according to Naidoo and Wills (2000), are an attempt to facilitate a 'bottom-up' approach to the provision of services with a greater focus on public health as opposed to acute services.

Creating supportive environments

The creation of a supportive environment by the nurse with other health care professionals can help to construct an atmosphere that is conducive to sexual health promotion. The environment in which the nurse sees his/her patients, i.e. the clinic, should be developed to meet local needs. The environment must be non-discriminatory, equitable and target population friendly, meaning – it must take into account the target population, e.g. gay men.

Nwokolo et al. (2002) describe how the views of young people had been taken into account when providing them with sexual health services. It was the young people who identified how they wanted the young person clinic to be set up. The nurse can influence and become involved in other care settings such as local youth clubs, outreach projects or prison services, with the aim of providing a helpful, caring environment for that particular client group.

Strengthening community action

Strengthening a community's ability to define their own health and service needs will ensure that the service provided is appropriate; this will mean that the nurse will usually have to become involved in working with and within a specific community group. The nurse may work in a variety of outreach projects; for example, working with commercial sex workers in their own environments, i.e. saunas, flats.

The aim would be to facilitate, enable and eventually empower the group to support and make decisions for themselves (Naidoo and Wills, 2000). The group might go on to address their own health needs and implement policy, both through and with their own community.

Developing personal skills

The nurse is ideally placed to develop and promote personal skills. By imparting skills and knowledge through health promotion activities, the patient may then be able to make informed, positive sexual health choices.

Interventions that focus upon, and emphasize, self-esteem acknowledge and recognize that the individual has a personal responsibility in adopting behaviours that may contribute to their quality of health. One example is the increased use of condoms after a community group has had facilitative interventions such as teaching and demonstrating the use of a condom. The facilitated intervention community group showed a significantly greater use of condoms than the control community group (the Centre for Disease Control and Prevention (CDC) AIDS Community Demonstration Projects Research Group, 1999).

In order for interventions to be successful and for individuals to develop personal skills – for example, in the use of condoms – then the material provided must be culturally appropriate and accessible. The information will need to be presented in a range of community languages, e.g. Urdu, Turkish (responding to the local target population).

Re-orienting services

A re-orientation or reframing of health services is needed if a health service is to meet the needs of its users. The focus has to move from the provision of care through a medical model to a more individual/patient-centred model. Potentially the medical model may have the ability to disempower the patient and as such this is antithetical to the philosophy underpinning health promotion (Scriven, 2001). The aim is to shift the balance of power from the medical establishment towards the patient, to facilitate access for those who may be disenfranchised. Services that offer more than an illness-based approach may provide better and more sustainable health outcomes for the users of those services. It is also important to acknowledge the substantial contribution made by other services, e.g. housing and economic developments, towards the promotion of health. Collaboration and intersectoral working are advocated in order to maximize the heath promoting potential of those services and for influencing the development and implementation of public policy.

To maximize sexual health and well-being, a planned and coordinated approach involving local multi-agency groups that is fully integrated across a range of services is advocated. Such an approach will need to ensure that action is taken to address local needs and that these activities are evidence based. Any activity related to health promotion will need to be ongoing and sustained: the nurse must therefore provide health promotion that has been thought about systematically and is based upon a model of health promotion (see Table 1.3).

Models of health promotion

Health promotion lies within the domain of clinical governance and is discussed not in isolation but in association with the fourteen components listed in Table 1.3.

There are several models of health promotion available that will help to deliver clinical governance. The explicit implementation of a model will enhance the overall function of the service. Colquhoun et al. (1997), Nutbeam (2000) and Colquhoun and Kellehear (1996) suggest that there are three main categories in which health promotion models can be placed:

- behavioural change model;
- self-empowerment model;
- collective action model.

Table 1.3 Fourteen components of clinical governance: health promotion is one of these components

Learning culture	Promoting and supporting a learning culture within the practice or workplace, e.g. primary, secondary and tertiary care
Research and development culture	Striving to produce practice that is evidence/research based
Reliable and accurate data	Basing nursing care and health promotion activities on reliable and accurate data
Well managed resources and services	Responding to local needs using both human and material resources appropriately. Identifying and working with other agencies
Coherent team	Ensuring that the team is well integrated and that staff from other agencies are also a part of that coherent team
Meaningful involvement of the public and the patient	Making sure that the local population has had its needs assessed and addressed. Making use of user groups, carers and expert patients, for example
Health gain	Devising and implementing activities that improve not only the health of the patient but also of staff
Confidentiality	Promoting an environment that adheres to the rules of confidentiality, emphasizing the importance of confidentiality
Policy and practice	Building and devising policy that is evidence based, striving to incorporate the activities of other agencies with an aim to provide joined up thinking and a seamless service
Accountability and performance	Adhering to the tenets of the NMC Code of Professional Conduct: Standards for Professional Conduct: Performance and Ethics (NMC, 2004a)
Core requirements	Measuring, monitoring and evaluating the performance of staff. Ongoing evaluation of services offered to ensure that staff are confident and competent. Consideration of skill mix and the numbers of staff required to provide the service
Health promotion	Devising ways and processes to promote health at every opportunity – opportunistic or planned interventions. Identifying those in most need and responding appropriately with materials that will begin to address their needs
Audit and evaluation	Ongoing evaluation – internally and by external agencies to determine if the provision is providing the most appropriate services
Risk management	Considering risk from the patient's perspective and also from a staff perspective

Adapted from Wakley and Chambers, 2002.

All three models and the elements associated with these models are not mutually exclusive; often all three are used together and interchangeably.

The behavioural change model

This model adopts a preventative approach and focuses on lifestyle behaviours that may influence health. The main thrust of this model is to persuade individuals to adopt healthy lifestyle behaviours/activities, to use preventative health care services and to take responsibility for their own health. This model has some positive aspects associated with it; however, it could be suggested that it employs a 'medical' model and that the issue of 'victim blaming' is inherent within it (Naidoo and Wills, 2000). One of the beliefs of this model is that if individuals are given the information (health promotion information) then this will encourage them to change their attitude, beliefs and behaviours. This model appears to neglect the other factors related to the way individuals act/behave; for example, the social environment the individual is a part of, the political forces at play, social, economic and cultural factors.

The self-empowerment model

Sometimes this model is known as the self-actualization model. Maslow (1954) refers to self-actualization in his hierarchy of needs. The characteristics of Maslow's 1954 model consider that an individual has a sense of reality, an awareness of real situations, is able to make objective judgements as opposed to subjective judgements, is democratic, fair and non-discriminatory – embracing and enjoying all cultures, races and individual styles.

The aim of the model is to enable and develop the individual in order to control their own health status as far as is possible, taking into account the effects of their environment. The notion of 'personal identity' is emphasized with this model as is 'self-worth', enhancing and developing the individual's 'life skills'. These life skills will include decision-making abilities and problem-solving skills, thus encouraging the individual to take control of their own life. This model, therefore, has as its key focus the individual; it is not targeted at groups.

Collective action model

This model is based on the view that health is influenced primarily by factors that function outside the control of the individual. It adopts a socio-ecological approach, taking into account the way in which the individual reacts/works with his/her environment – the interrelationship between the two. The Ottawa Charter (WHO, 1986) advocated that health promotion activity should embrace an approach that uses a socio-ecological approach. This approach will then encourage those who provide health promotion to consider how people and their environments are inextricably linked.

The model believes that community empowerment and commitment is key, suggesting that the people – individually and collectively – will acquire the knowledge, understanding and skills to improve societal structures that have a powerful effect on people's health status. The idea underpinning this model is that critical thinking needs to take place that will engage the collective to act and contribute positively (Health Development Agency, 2000). This model has the potential to achieve healthy outcomes for both individuals and groups in society through a participative approach. Table 1.4 considers the characteristics of health promotion and health education models.

Table 1.4 Characteristics of health promotion and health education models

Behavioural change model
- Emphasis on the nurses' perception of health needs – a medical model approach with paternalistic overtones – 'nurse knows best'
- Has the ability to provide knowledge, thus increasing the individual's knowledge base related to the improvement and enhancement of health
- Educates about health
- Sees the patient as a passive participant in the transmission of knowledge
- Encourages the idea that health is solely an individual's concern/responsibility – 'healthism'
- Could be seen as 'moralistic'
- Emphasizes the disease process
- Focuses on risk as opposed to prevention
- Can neglect the socio-ecological perspective
- Has the ability to imply 'victim blaming'

Self-empowerment model
- Promotes and develops a sense of identity
- Encourages the individual to consider self in relation to society
- Encourages independence
- Emphasizes the need for critical thinking and action
- Considers individual action and emphasizes determinants that may be beyond their control
- Promotes resilience and empowerment at a personal level as opposed to a collective level
- Enhances self-awareness
- Allows the celebration of individuality

Collective action model

- Sees the patient and the nurse as social agents
- Emphasizes a patient centred approach, i.e. recognizes and values the contribution made by the patient
- Uses a whole community approach as opposed to an individual approach
- Includes and takes into consideration the determinants of health
- Empowers all participants
- Educates for health – promotes health
- Uses social action to engineer work with others
- Participation by all for all is emphasized
- Accepts that a holistic inclusive approach is appropriate
- Empowers all participants

Source: adapted from Nutbeam, 2000; Colquhoun et al., 1997.

Table 1.5 demonstrates ways in which the three models may be used in the context of health promotion and the use of condoms.

Table 1.5 Some ways in which all three models may be used to increase the use of condoms

Behavioural change model

- Use of slogans
- Media messages
- Pamphlets

Self-empowerment model

- Provision of access to free condoms and lubricant
- Provision of help lines/websites for confidential advice giving
- Support groups in targeted populations, e.g. the gay community

Collective action model

- Working with specific groups, e.g. gay men, adolescents
- Engaging with these specific groups to determine and identify needs
- Developing policy and support structures with members of the specific groups

Seedhouse (1986) suggests that health is the foundation for all achievement. He points out that the idea that health is particular, precisely determined and a fully informed structure that each individual can achieve is preposterous. There is no such thing, he continues, as a faultless person. The foundations theory of health promotion has been postulated by Seedhouse (1997). The key supposition is the extent to which a person's autonomy reflects his/her health status. The foundations for health need to be in place prior to the person being in a position to attain optimal health. Watkinson (2002) provides a simplified version of Seedhouse's (1997) foundations for health theory (see Figure 1.3).

Basic needs fulfilled	Key information available	Ability to understand and 'do'	Community integration	Bonus or supportive box
1	2	3	4	5

Figure 1.3 The foundations theory of health promotion. Source: Watkinson, 2002.

Watkinson (2002) suggests that a person will enjoy a high level of health if all aspects of the first four boxes have been achieved or are available, with the fifth box being called into play as and when necessary. If the contents of any of the first four boxes are missing then the person will have or experience a lower level of health.

Preparing health promotion materials

This section of the chapter offers the reader some guidance for the preparation of written patient information. The quality of information presented to patients can influence each experience they have with health care provision and providers (DoH, 2003c). The importance of improving information that is given to patients has been cited in some key government publications, for example the NHS Plan (DoH, 2000a), Kennedy Report into the Bristol Royal Infirmary (2001) and Good Practice in Consent (DoH, 2001b).

Often nurses may need to provide patients with information concerning their condition, treatment, investigation, examination procedures and services available; this may be in the form of leaflets, posters, or a single sheet of paper. Attention to the information provided is important as it can instil confidence in patients, remind them of what is happening or what is going to happen and allow them to make informed decisions.

The principles underpinning good patient communication are to:

- improve health;
- provide the best care;
- act professionally;
- work efficiently;
- treat everybody equally (DoH, 2003c).

The written information provided to patients can support these values and the following should be taken into account. Communication should be:

- clear – so it can be understood;
- straightforward – using fewer words keeping to the necessary information;
- modern – using everyday language and current images;
- accessible – available to as many people as possible, avoiding jargon, up to date;
- honest – based on current evidence;
- respectful – sensitive to cultural needs and avoiding stereotypes.

When providing information the nurse needs to take into account who it is intended for and what the purpose is. It is advocated that the nurse writes from the patient's perspective, assuming that the patient has little knowledge of what is being communicated. There may be situations when this is inappropriate, for example, when communicating with 'expert' patients – patients who have a long-term medical condition.

When the information has been written, the nurse needs to decide how best to present it. The more clear, inviting and high-quality the product is the more likely people are to read it. It is always important to proofread the proposed publication prior to printing. Large print may be needed for those who have eyesight difficulties, Braille may be needed or they may need the provision of audio tapes. For children, illustrations may enhance the message being given. Those patients who have a learning disability may benefit from information that has been simplified, using symbols and pictures; the nurse should consult support groups to determine the most appropriate format – and should avoid patronizing the patient. For those patients whose first language is not English the text will need to be translated from a guaranteed source. Audio tapes and videos may be used for those patients who have reading problems.

Table 1.6 provides a checklist of issues that should be considered when putting together a leaflet or booklet. This is not a complete checklist and not all of the items will be relevant; it is meant only as a guide.

Table 1.6 Checklist outlining items that should be considered by the nurse when formulating leaflets and booklets for operations, treatments and investigations

- What is the leaflet about and who is it for?
- What is the procedure?
- Why are they having it? (Give the benefits and alternatives where appropriate)
- What preparation do they need or not need?
- Do they need a general anaesthetic, sedation or local anaesthetic?
- What happens when they arrive at the hospital/clinic/surgery, who will meet them?

Table 1.6 continued

- Will they be asked to sign a consent form or is verbal consent needed?
- What does the procedure involve? How long does it last? What does it feel like?
- What happens after the procedure – pain control, nursing checks, e.g. observations, stitches?
- How long will they be at the hospital/clinic/surgery?
- Do they need someone with them or any special equipment when they get home?
- What care do they need at home?
- What follow-up care is needed? Do they need to visit their doctor?
- What can go wrong, what signs to look out for and what to do if something goes wrong?
- When can they start their normal activities again, for example, driving, sport, sex or work?
- Who can they contact if they have any more questions?
- Tell people where they can find more information, for example, support groups and websites

Source: adapted from DoH, 2003c.

Table 1.7 provides a checklist for information to be given to patients concerning their condition and treatment.

Table 1.7 A checklist for information to be given to patients concerning their condition and treatment

- What is the leaflet about and who is it for?
- What condition is being described?
- What causes it? Or, if the cause is not known say so
- Does anything increase the risk, for example age, sex, ethnic origin or a family history of the condition?
- What are the signs and symptoms?
- Are there any tests or examinations needed to confirm the diagnosis?
- What treatments are available? Give brief descriptions
- What are the side effects and the risks of getting treatment or not getting treatment?
- What are the next steps?
- What can patients do for themselves?
- Are there other implications, for example, infecting other people?
- Who can they contact if they have more questions?
- Say where the patient can find more information, for example, support groups and websites

Source: DoH, 2003c.

Conclusion

There are many definitions of the term 'health' available to the nurse and some of these have been discussed. Health is a complex concept; it is dynamic and in a constant state of flux. Sexual health also has its own dimensions and is best seen when set in context. This chapter has provided the reader with an overview of the dynamics associated with health promotion and has examined three particular models of health promotion: the self-empowerment model, behavioural change model and collective action model. The models, when applied to practice, are not mutually exclusive and often they are used together and interchangeably. The underlying difference with each model is the philosophical framework that they have adopted. Examples have been cited related to the use of condoms using all three different models.

One key health provision framework, the Ottawa Charter, has been discussed; this framework is well suited to sexual health care delivery as it aims to bring about positive long-term changes to the health of communities. The framework has five strategies: developing personal skills, creating supportive environments, strengthening community action, building healthy public policy and re-orienting services in the interest of health. This framework allows a collaborative intersectoral approach to be developed in order to maximize the individual's health potential. Health promotion activity must take into account influences at local, national and international levels:

- local level – responding to local need, e.g. HiMPs;
- national level – national strategy, e.g. Sexual Health Strategy;
- international level – global projects, e.g. WHO initiatives.

In order to communicate effectively, it is important that the nurse carefully considers the ways in which health promotion messages are conveyed, e.g. leaflets or booklets. Some of the principles underpinning good patient communication are: to improve health, provide the best care, act professionally, work effectively and treat everybody equally. The final aspect of the chapter offers suggestions for developing health promotion materials and a checklist is provided.

CHAPTER TWO

The sexual health history

Introduction

High quality sexual health history taking and risk assessment can provide opportunities for targeted sexual health promotion to become a routine part of good patient care. Obtaining a sexual health history can be a part of general history taking; it does not lie within the sole province of the sexual health nurse. Nurses in various settings may encounter patients who have diseases or psychological conditions that have a direct correlation with their recent or past sexual behaviour. The outcomes of the sexual health history can also enable people to receive appropriately targeted advice and information on prevention of STIs, HIV or unintended pregnancies within the clinical setting (Medical Foundation for Sexual Health, 2004). The sexual health history, therefore, is not only about gaining information to detect if the patient has an STI; but is also about the patient's sexual well-being, their entirety.

The accuracy of the information collected from a patient during the course of an STI can significantly influence the diagnosis and subsequent treatment; therefore, taking a competent history is crucial to the patient encounter and patient outcome (Matthews, 1998).

Johnson et al. (2002) have noted in their study related to sexual attitudes and lifestyles that there has been an increase in risky sexual behaviour. This finding may mean that health care providers will have to reconsider their role in promoting sexual health (Verhoeven et al., 2003). Valuable opportunities exist for nurses to raise the issue of STIs and to address sexual health concerns when undertaking a sexual health history.

Society appears to adopt an unclear outlook in relation to sex in spite of the candid presence of sexuality in the media. Johnson et al. (2002) suggest that many people, including nurses and doctors, regard sexual issues as 'personal', even when these issues are within the confines of health care settings. It has been identified that the discussion of sexual matters is difficult to talk about with patients (Tomlinson, 1998). Furthermore, Haley et al. (1999) note that within the primary health care setting STI counselling is hardly ever carried out and this is often deficient.

There has been a shift towards asymptomatic STIs such as chlamydial and gonoccocal infection (Low et al., 2003; Verhoeven et al., 2003). This may provoke more potential problems for the nurse in raising the issue of STI with his/her patients. Patients may not present with any complaints, and as such may not have even considered the issue of an STI despite the possibility of being infected with one (Matthews and Fletcher, 2001). Taking a sexual health history demands a skilled, confident and competent nurse and this chapter will examine this important activity in detail.

Record-keeping

Almost every encounter the nurse has with the patient will inevitably involve recording the information that has been exchanged between the two parties. The nurse must adhere to local policy pertaining to records and record-keeping. The NMC (2004b) provide guidelines for records and record-keeping. Record-keeping is a fundamental aspect of nurses', midwives' and specialist community public health nurses' professional practice. Whilst the NMC (2004b) provide guidance they do not dictate the content, nor do they provide a rigid framework for the content of records or record-keeping. As individually accountable practitioners, the nurse, midwife and community public health nurse are expected to exercise their professional judgement. Good record-keeping, according to the NMC (2004b), helps to protect the interests of the patient by promoting:

- high standards of clinical care;
- continuity of care;
- better communication and dissemination of information between members of the interprofessional health care team;
- an accurate account of treatment, care planning and delivery;
- the ability to detect problems, such as a change in the patient's condition, at an early stage.

The documentation used to detail the sexual health history will need to be decided at a local level with other members of the interprofessional health care team, as there is no one model or template available.

There are many components associated with record-keeping, e.g. style and content. One other factor that also needs to be taken into consideration is the legal implications that the nurse needs to be aware of; Table 2.1 outlines some of these facets.

Table 2.1 Factors that can contribute to effective record-keeping

Patient records should:
- be factual, consistent and accurate
- be written as soon as possible after an event has occurred, providing current information on the care and condition of the patient
- be written clearly and in such a manner that the text cannot be erased
- be written in such a manner that any alterations or additions are dated, timed and signed in such a way that the original entry can still be read clearly
- be accurately dated, timed and signed, with the signature printed alongside the first entry
- not include abbreviations, jargon, meaningless phrases, irrelevant speculation and offensive subjective statements
- be readable on any photocopies
- be written whenever possible with the involvement of the patient
- be written in terms that the patient can understand
- be consecutive
- identify problems that have arisen and the actions that have been taken to rectify them
- provide clear evidence of the care planned, the decisions made, the care delivered and the information shared

Source: adapted from NMC, 2004b.

There are occasions when patient records may be called as evidence before a court of law by the Health Service Commissioner, or at a local level, to investigate a complaint. The Nursing and Midwifery Council may also ask for records to be called for when the Fitness to Practise Committees are investigating complaints made about nurses, midwives and community public health nurses. Records in this instance may include:

- care plans;
- diaries;
- anything that makes reference to the patient.

Records should be able to demonstrate that the nurse has acted professionally and in the best interests of the patient (see Table 2.2).

Courts of law may approach record-keeping by suggesting that 'if it is not recorded, it has not been done'. Under judicial examination the nursing record will determine your professional credibility if your memory fades (Epstein et al., 1997). The nurse has to exercise her/his professional judgement as to what is relevant, what is to be recorded and the frequency of entries (Fletcher and Buka, 1999). Errors do occur in record-keeping and Table 2.3 highlights some of these.

Good record-keeping can result in good communications but the message being communicated will only be as good as the nurse who is

Table 2.2 Aspects of documentation which demonstrate that the nurse has taken into account their duty of care to the patient within a professional framework

The record should demonstrate:
• A full account of the assessment, the care planned and what has been implemented
• Relevant information about the patient's condition at any given time and any measures that have been taken in response to patient needs
• Evidence that the nurse has understood and honoured the duty of care owed to the patient, that all reasonable tasks have been taken to care for the patient and that any actions or omissions have not compromised patient safety in any way
• A record of any arrangements that the nurse has made for the continuing care of the patient

Source: adapted from NMC, 2004b.

Table 2.3 Some common errors noted in patient records

• Time omitted
• Illegible handwriting
• Abbreviations were ambiguous
• Use of correction fluid to cover up errors
• No signature
• Inaccuracies, especially of the dates
• Delay in completing the record; in some cases more than 24 hours had elapsed before the record was completed
• Inaccuracies of name, date of birth and address
• Unprofessional terminology, e.g. 'dull as a door step'
• Meaningless phrases, e.g. 'lovely child'
• Opinion mixed up with facts
• Subjective not objective comments, e.g. 'normal development'

Source: adapted from Dimond, 2005.

recording the information. Other colleagues may rely on the information contained in your records and as a result may act on what has been recorded. Each registered nurse, midwife and community public health nurse must be aware that they are professionally accountable for any duties they delegate to any other member of the interprofessional health care team. This includes the delegation of record-keeping to pre-registration nursing and midwifery students or health care assistants. It is imperative that these members of the team are adequately supervised and that they are competent to carry out the task. The nurse should countersign any such entry and remember that they are professionally accountable for the consequences of such an entry. The NMC (2004b) would strongly advise that initials should not be used; the full signature should be used with the name written alongside it. Good record-keeping is the hallmark of a skilled, competent, confident and safe practitioner.

The sexual health history

The sexual health history is taken in order to discover the problems the patient may have with their sexuality or with an STI. It is the role of the nurse to ascertain the reason for the consultation; otherwise the problem may remain unresolved, resulting in further problems for the patient or their sexual partners (Wakley et al., 2003). It also has another use: it is often the key document used in audit, to assess quality control in nursing practice.

From the outset the nurse should discuss with patients what will be written in the notes and how the information will be managed, for example, information concerning risk behaviour (Curtis et al., 1995). Being open and honest about the importance of gathering information and documenting it while emphasizing that the team have a commitment to confidentiality may reassure the patient that the information collected will be treated with respect, kept safe and when disclosure is to be made to a third party this will be done with their consent and will be made in their best interests.

Gaining consent from the patient to undertake the sexual health history may be implicit in the nurse–patient relationship; the patient also needs permission to divulge and discuss intimate details. The PLISSIT model (Annon, 1975) provides a framework for the patient and the nurse to approach sexual concerns (see Table 2.4).

Table 2.4 The PLISSIT model for approaching sexual health problems

Permission:
This is the first step and is essential; by asking the patient for permission to discuss sexual matters the nurse is showing respect and sensitivity towards the patient. It could also be suggested at this juncture that the patient is giving permission to discuss sexuality now and in the future. Permission may also be given to the patient to continue with what it is they are doing sexually; it is an assurance that their sexual behaviours and fantasies are acceptable or 'normal'. The nurse must guard against giving permission to the patient to engage in or continue to engage in activities that are potentially harmful to him/herself or others

Limited information:
This aspect of the framework allows the patient and the nurse to clarify misinformation, dispel myths and provide factual information in a limited manner. By giving limited information the nurse should not be prescribing sexual practices for the patient but should be providing information that the patient may choose to use or not

Table 2.4 continued

Specific suggestion:
The nurse can provide specific information to the patient allowing the patient to consider their problem. Providing the patient with suggestions for them to work through to continue with their sexual relations empowers the patient

Intensive treatment:
This aspect of the framework comes into play when the patient's case is complex and may require highly individualized therapy or referral for the complex issues

Source: adapted from Annon, 1975.

Epstein et al. (1997) suggest that it is the history that guides the patient through a series of questions designed to build a profile of the patient and their sexual problems. The history culminates in the nurse having a deeper understanding of the patient and differential diagnosis may have been arrived at, explaining the symptoms the patient has presented with.

The range of questions asked, adopting a holistic approach, will range from the presenting symptoms to:

- the social history;
- education;
- employment history;
- personal habits;
- psycho-social history;
- travel;
- home circumstances;
- family history;
- sexual history/activity;
- a review of the major organs.

Nusbaum and Hamilton (2002) suggest that by increasing the number of times the sexual health history is taken, and the number of times enquiries of a sexual health nature occur, this may subsequently improve sexual health and well-being by identifying as early as possible any sexual problems. Incorporating sexual health history taking into the usual/routine history-taking exercise can provide opportunities for the nurse to offer preventative care such as immunization against hepatitis B and counselling opportunities related to risk minimizing sexual behaviours.

When doctors in one study increased their sexual history-taking frequency, it was noted that the rate of sexual health problems reported by their patients increased sixfold (Bachmann et al., 1989). Similar results may also be evident when the nurse increases his/her enquiries regarding sexual health: the more the nurse incorporates sexual health history taking into the usual/routine history taking activities, the more competent he/she will become in conducting them.

It is important that the nurse incorporates sexual health history taking into the general consultation process, to see it as an integral aspect of the assessment process. The nurse must adopt a holistic approach; identifying problems at an early stage can have implications for morbidity and mortality. For example chlamydia has fertility and neonatal complications associated with it, and the human papillomavirus brings with it the risk of pre-invasive and invasive lower genital tract disease. Maurice and Bowman (1999) state that the morbidity and mortality caused by HIV and STIs are significant. Early recognition and treatment of these conditions can have a significant impact on positive outcomes.

The sexual health history can also reveal the prevalence of sexual dysfunction experienced by the patient and his/her partner. Sexual dysfunction difficulties associated with sexual function and concerns regarding sex are common. Goldmeier et al. (2000) demonstrate that there are a substantial proportion of attenders at a central London genitourinary medicine clinic who have sexual dysfunction; this may lead to both psychological and physical problems.

Problems with sexual dysfunction as a result of medications or surgical interventions can also be revealed by an in-depth sexual health history. Side effects may occur as a result of prescribed medication, for example antidepressants, or the result of surgical intervention, such as a trans-urethral resection of the prostate gland. By becoming aware of these problems the nurse can make a request for a review of the medications or offer support and provide appropriate referral.

While obtaining a sexual health history the nurse may determine the reason for current health problems the patient may be experiencing. Anxiety/depression, for example, may be the consequences of sexual abuse experienced by the patient either recently, currently or in the past.

Wilson and McAndrew (2000) state that high quality care provision means incorporating sexual health into all aspects of patient care and as such it should be seen to be as important as the physical, spiritual, social and emotional aspects of care. Bachmann et al. (1989) suggest that with this in mind it should be just as natural to ask about sexual orientation as it is to ask the patient about bowel habits.

Some nurses may be proficient at conducting and obtaining a standard history from a patient but they may lack confidence in dealing with a history that focuses upon the patient's sexual health. Wakley et al. (2003) outline some reasons why discomfort may arise when starting to talk to patients about sex:

• fear of offending the patient;

- unfamiliarity with the patient's culture (either their ethnicity or sexual orientation);
- unwillingness to become involved in complex and time-consuming issues;
- reticence and embarrassment.

The patient may also be reluctant to speak out about sex because of:

- embarrassment, shame or humiliation;
- unease about their sexuality;
- concerns about the information being given and confidentiality;
- the presence of a partner;
- worries about being judged inadequate or odd.

If the nurse fails to take a sexual health history this could be tantamount to professional misconduct as it may breach the truism 'to do no harm' or 'to act in the patient's best interests'. Nusbaum and Hamilton (2002) provide an example of this – if a patient presents with multiple episodes of cervicitis and is never asked about her sexual health, e.g. her sexual behaviour, or is never provided with information regarding the risks of having multiple partners and the association between this and an increased risk of human papillomavirus and cervical cancer, then she has not received optimal health care – her needs, it could be suggested, have been neglected.

Sexual activity and lifestyles – what is the 'norm'?

Sexual activity and what society considers is the 'norm' will vary from individual to individual and from culture to culture. In the past there has been little reliable information on sexual behaviour in the United Kingdom; however, surveys such as the National Survey of Sexual Attitudes and Lifestyles (NATSAL, 2000) have provided more data on reported sexual behaviours. The Family Planning Association (FPA) (2003) suggests that there has been a significant change in the public's awareness and social attitudes towards HIV/AIDS and STIs, all of which may have influenced sexual behaviour.

The average age at first intercourse has fallen from 17 years to 16 years for both males and females since the 1990s; approximately 25 per cent of men and 30 per cent of women aged 16 to 19 years first had sexual intercourse before the age of 16 years. Wellings et al. (2001) state that the proportion of women reporting first intercourse before 16 years increased up to, but not after, the mid-1990s. Early age at first intercourse was significantly associated with pregnancy under 18 years, but not with occurrence of STIs.

The following results are reported by Johnson et al. (2002) concerning partnerships and practices, and patterns of heterosexual and homosexual partnership varied substantially by age, residence in Greater London, and marital status. In the past five years, mean numbers of heterosexual partners were 3.8 for men, and 2.4 for women; 2.6 per cent of both men and women reported homosexual partnerships; and 4.3 per cent of men reported paying for sex.

It is estimated that 14 per cent of men and 13 per cent of women have reported anal intercourse in heterosexual encounters; as anal intercourse is often seen as immoral or taboo, these figures may be under-representations. Three-quarters of women and 70 per cent of men have experienced oral sex at some time, and masturbation – a common activity – is reported by 66 per cent of women and 99 per cent of men.

The NATSAL (2000) survey demonstrated that 8.3 per cent of men in their survey had had a sexual experience, not necessarily including genital contact, with a partner of the same sex, 6.3 per cent had had sex with a same sex partner, including genital contact; for women these figures were 9.7 per cent and 5.7 per cent respectively.

Interviewing techniques and sexual history taking

Taking a sexual health history requires the same skills as other history taking; there are, however, other additional difficulties associated with sexual health history (Wakley and Chambers, 2002). The interview is the main point of the nurse–patient relationship and this confirms the bond between the two parties, in order to begin to provide care for the patient. Taking and recording a competent sexual health history is key to the clinical process (Carter et al., 1998).

Asking the patient questions about sexual function and practice can be life-saving; good interviewing techniques can help to prevent risks associated with life-threatening STIs and HIV (Bickley and Szilagyi, 2003).

It is important that the nurse conveys the message that it is safe to talk about sexual behaviour and sexuality, as this is normal during any consultation. Using a calm but sensitive manner will place the nurse and the patient in an advantageous position.

There are no hard and fast rules of taking a sexual health history: every nurse will have his/her own way of dealing with sexual health matters. A comfortable atmosphere with a relaxed, but professional and friendly, approach is what the nurse should be aiming to create. The manner in which the interview is conducted will impinge on the amount of information the patient is prepared to reveal. The nurse must establish rapport and trust with the patient, acknowledging that many people find it difficult to talk about sexually related matters (French, 2004a). Some patients may present their problems in disguise or use euphemisms, innuendo and non-verbal signs to describe their problems, as they may fear being criticized, judged or condemned about their reason for attendance. Revealing intimate, personal and potentially embarrassing information may be difficult for the patient; therefore the nurse needs to be able to provide a safe environment in which to do this.

The setting

The patient (in some instances with his/her partner) may be interviewed in a variety of settings, e.g. on the open ward, in the out-patients' department, in the GP surgery, in the clinic or even in their own home. Noise and interruptions can be disconcerting and cause distraction; if possible a quiet room should be sought in which to conduct the interview.

Seating and the way this has been arranged are important considerations. The patient's seat should be placed in such a way as to avoid the use of a desk as this may appear confrontational: place the seats at the side of the desk. This gives the nurse an opportunity to observe the patient's body language. It must not be forgotten that this type of arrangement also allows the patient to observe the nurse's body language. Observations on body language are considered in Table 2.5.

Table 2.5 Observations on body language

- Use of hands and arms, for example, uneasy twiddling with ring or bracelet, crossing of arms in a defensive manner, holding up a bag or briefcase as if for protection
- A pectoral flush that sweeps over the upper chest and neck possibly indicating a feeling of unease regardless of a confident outward appearance
- Position in the chair, i.e. slumped back onto the chair, sitting tautly erect or a relaxed sprawl
- When there is harmony and a sense of empathy between the two (patient and nurse) a postural echo may be adopted, for example when the nurse and the patient sit in mirror image of each other's position

Source: adapted from Tomlinson, 1998.

Time

The timing of the interview is important: avoid meal times or rest periods. There must be sufficient time set aside by the nurse, and when possible the patient should be told how long will be needed to conduct an in-depth interview. Tomlinson (1998) suggests that between 45 and 60 minutes will be needed.

Promoting comfort

It has already been stated that a matter of fact approach may encourage the patient to feel safe, relax and talk openly. The patient may divulge information that the nurse finds shocking; however, it is imperative that a non-judgemental approach is taken. Nurses often use techniques to promote comfort intuitively. This is evidenced by the way they greet the patient, ensuring the patient is comfortable with the seating arrangements and ensuring privacy. A 'do not disturb' sign may need to be used on office doors, telephones should be diverted and mobile telephones should be switched off to minimize disturbances.

Most employers provide badges for the nurse to wear to identify them; however, this should never prevent you from introducing yourself to the patient, explaining to them who you are and the purpose of the encounter. It is important to determine how the patient would like to be referred to – on a first-name basis or by a more formal title. The nurse must also take into consideration how s/he is dressed for the interview; some units may have a dress code/policy. Epstein et al. (1997) suggest that the way the health care professional is dressed can have implications for the relationship between the nurse and the patient.

Questions to ask and issues to raise

It may help the patient if the nurse explains the reason why such personal questions are being asked. For example, 'I am asking these types of questions so that I can assess your needs fully and work out the right tests for you, therefore I need to know a bit more detail about your sex life.'

When the nurse approaches the sexual history taking exercise as if asking questions from a questionnaire or a list to be run through with the patient, this will lose all of its potential worth. If the nurse asks a lot of questions then the patient will give a lot of answers. However, the problem s/he has been presented with may not have been identified because the nurse has not allowed the patient the time to talk. The nurse must listen to the patient and use silence if need be to allow or give the patient permission to tell their story. Effective communication skills are paramount; the use of open-ended questions, for example, which do not necessitate a yes/no response, is advocated in order to elicit as much information as possible (Carter et al., 1998). Examples of open, closed and judgemental questions are cited in Table 2.6.

It has already been recognized that some patients present their problems in disguise or use euphemisms, innuendo and non-verbal signs; they are often circumlocutory, and as this is the case the nurse has to attempt to determine what they are trying to say and to clarify what was said.

Table 2.6 Some examples of open, closed and judgemental questions

Open questions:
'How can I help you?'
'What is the problem?'
'What do you think caused the difficulty?'

Closed questions:
'Did you use a condom?'
'Have you had this kind of discharge before?'
'Does it hurt after you have had intercourse?'

Judgemental questions:
'At your age don't you think you should know better?'
'As a health care professional you, of all people, should have known better'

Source: adapted from Tomlinson, 1998.

Tomlinson (1998) suggests that words used by men, for example 'impotence', may mean different things to different men and their partners – failing to achieve an erection, failure to maintain an erection and premature ejaculation. Phrases such as 'I am sore down below' can mean many things – for example, anything from pruritis ani to a prolapse or genital herpes. The nurse's role is to elucidate and clarify carefully and tactfully.

The nurse should avoid using terms that make assumptions either about the patient's sexual behaviour or their sexuality. When asking about a patient's sexual orientation it is advised that the nurse uses the term 'partner' as opposed to 'boyfriend' or 'girlfriend', 'husband' or 'wife'. Ask about how many partners the patient has instead of asking if they are married and/or monogamous. The response the patient gives to how many partners they have may confirm if they are married and monogamous.

When discussing sexual behaviour the nurse must make certain that the patient understands the terminology being used; failing to do this may render the whole exercise worthless. The nurse may be concerned about bringing vernacular terms into the consultation because of embarrassment and the patient may avoid using colloquialisms as they may fear causing offence. The nurse needs to decide, in order to avoid confusion and misinterpretation, if s/he will use street talk and/or colloquialisms, and thereby potentially forfeit professionalism. There are no hard and fast rules here, and often the line is fine and is associated with the age and gender of both the patient and nurse.

Conducting the interview with the patient alone or with the partner present needs much deliberation. The patient may not be as forthcoming with information if the partner is present; however, joint consultations can provide much important detail. The nurse will need to exercise his/her professional judgement in coming to a decision.

To obtain a complete sexual health history the nurse will need to consider the patient's social and medical history and the problem must be seen from the patient's perspective. The following points can be addressed:

- How long has the problem been present?
- Is it related to a particular time, place, or partner?
- Does the problem cause a loss of sex drive or any dislike of sexual contact?
- Do you have any problems in your relationship?
- Are there any physical problems experienced, such as pain, felt either by yourself or your partner?

When considering the patient's social history, the nurse will be able to place the patient into context. Asking the patient about family life (and the term family is how the patient defines it), home and job – familiar things – can give both the nurse and the patient time to relax.

Assessing medical history, current and past, can help the nurse and the patient understand some problems they may be experiencing. Table 2.7 outlines some medical conditions that can have an effect on the patient's sexual heath and well-being.

Table 2.7 Some medical conditions that may have an effect on the patient's sexual health and well-being

Diabetes mellitus
Diabetes mellitus may result in impotence in nearly fifty percent of men affected

Other hormonal diseases
Abnormalities with thyroid and testosterone can reduce sexual desire and performance in both men and women

Mental health difficulties
Depressive illnesses and psychotic problems can cause loss of libido in a high proportion of both men and women

Surgery and trauma
Gynaecological and prostatic surgery, in particular, can create sexual health problems; surgery within the abdomen, e.g. stoma formation, may also lead to loss of libido and erectile difficulties. Trauma to the pelvis or spine is also implicated in sexual dysfunction experienced by men and women

Cardiac disease
Erectile dysfunction is associated with heart disease, hyperlipidaemia and arteriopathy in men. Post-myocardial infarction and cardiac surgery can have an effect upon the

Table 2.7 continued

quality of sexual health, fear and anxiety concerning the resumption of sexual activity after the event causing many people to postpone or not resume sexual activity

Pain
Many types of pain experienced by the patient can impair their quality of sexual health, for example cardiac pain, arthritic pain, phimosis or vaginismus

Prescribed and recreational drugs
Numerous drugs – prescribed or recreational – can result in sexual dysfunction, for example:

• Anticonvulsants
• Antidepressants
• Antipsychotics
• Antihypertensives
• Diuretics
• Anti-emetics
• Non-steroidal anti-inflammatories
• Anticholinergics
• Antispasmodics
• Barbiturates
• Cannabis
• Alcohol

Source: adapted from Tomlinson, 1998; Wakley and Chambers, 2002; Wakley et al., 2003.

Once the nurse has taken an in-depth sexual health history the next step, with the patient, is to decide on a way forward, to address and treat the problem. Chapter 3 discusses the management of some common STIs.

Obtaining a sexual health history from children, young people and people with learning disabilities may be challenging as the carer or parents may have accompanied the patient and may tend to answer for the patient; the patient may also be reluctant to divulge information with a third party present. The use of dolls, puppets and images to demonstrate what is being discussed can help. Wakley et al. (2003) advocate breaking each period of communication/interaction into shorter parts, checking after each section that all parties understand what is being said. The nurse needs to be aware of his/her limitations and be prepared to refer the patient to a more appropriate health care professional if s/he is feeling out of his/her depth.

A checklist of questions

Table 2.8 is a checklist to help you conduct the sexual health history with confidence. It includes issues that you may find appropriate and some that you may find inappropriate; as time goes by and the more sexual health histories you take, the more proficient you will become. The way the questions are asked and the terminology used will depend on your assessment of the patient's understanding. This checklist should be used as an aide mémoire to help guide the consultation.

Table 2.8 Checklist of questions that may help guide and inform the sexual health history

General issues:
- Are you currently sexually active?
- Do you have any worries about your sex life?
- Do you have more than one sexual partner?
- Do you have sex with men, women or both?
- Tell me about your sexual activity. For example, do you have oral/anal sex?
- Do you masturbate?
- Are you sexually satisfied?
- Is your sexual activity as frequent as you would like it to be?
- Does your partner prefer more or less sexual activity than you do?
- Do you have orgasms?
- Is there any pain associated with sexual activity – you/your partner?
- Is there anything about your sexual activity that you would want to change?
- Do you have any worries about your genitals?

Menstrual and obstetric issues:
- At what age did menstruation begin?
- When did you have your last menstrual period?
- Have you ever had unprotected intercourse, if so when and how often?
- About your periods:
  - How long do they last?
  - Are/were they regular?
  - How often did/do they occur?
- Do/did you ever have pain, bleeding or discomfort during your period or during intercourse?
- Do you experience any problems with premenstrual syndrome?
- Do you experience any menopausal symptoms (offer examples)?
- Have you ever had any pregnancy related problems (offer examples)?

Pregnancy intentions (these questions should be directed at both the man and the woman):
- Do you plan to have a child, if so how soon would you like to become a parent?
- Do you need any advice on getting pregnant or on care during pregnancy?
- Do you have any worries about your fertility?
- If pregnancy is not an intention just now, are you and your partner taking precautions or any forms of protection from pregnancy?

Table 2.8 continued

STIs:

- Have you ever had an STI?
- Do you think you are at risk of getting an STI?
- How many sexual partners have you had in the last 12 months?
- Have you ever experienced a burning sensation when you pass water?
- Have you had any discharge from your genitalia?
- Have you had any rash or lumps in the genital area?

Prostatic issues:

- When passing urine have you had any dribbling?
- Do you feel the urge to pass water frequently?
- Do you have to get up in the night to pass urine?
- Have you noticed any reduction in the flow of your urine?
- Do you experience any lower abdominal pain?
- Do you have pain on ejaculation?

Hepatitis:

- Have you ever had a yellowing of the skin or eyes, or have any of your friends told you that you look yellow?
- Have you ever had:
  - Upper abdominal pain?
  - Light coloured stools?
  - Dark urine?
- Have you ever been told you have a liver problem or hepatitis?
- Have you ever been vaccinated for hepatitis?

Alcohol and drug use:

- How many alcoholic drinks do you have each day – beer, wine, spirit?
- Is alcohol or drug use interfering with your life?
- Does your use of alcohol/drugs concern you, your friends or family?
- Have you ever got in trouble because of drug or alcohol use?

Medication:

- What prescribed medications are you currently taking?
- What over the counter medications are you currently taking?
- Are you taking any herbs, vitamins or supplements – what are they?

Physical, sexual and emotional issues:

- When young, did anyone ever touch you in a way that made you feel uncomfortable?
- When young, did anyone ever ask you to, or make you, touch their body in a sexual way?
- Has anyone ever hit or battered you?
- Do you live with anyone who verbally abuses you?
- Have you ever been forced to have sex against your will?

Table 2.8 continued

Medical or surgical trauma:
- Have you ever had any injuries or surgery to your genitals or genital area?
- Have you had a vasectomy?
- Have you had a hysterectomy?
- Are you sterilized?
- If you have had children, were the deliveries normal?
- Have you ever been treated with radiotherapy or chemotherapy?
- Have you any worries or concerns about your genitals?

Source: Wakley et al., 2003; Epstein et al., 1997; Nusbaum and Hamilton, 2002.

Conclusion

Taking a comprehensive sexual health history is the key to good sexual health care. The nurse needs to continue to develop and hone his/her sexual history taking skills in order to become confident with this often complex and emotive skill. One aspect of respect towards the patient is respecting his/her decision or reluctance not to disclose all sexual relationship details.

There are barriers to obtaining an in-depth sexual health history and these can impinge on the quality of data with which the patient provides the nurse, in order to plan and implement subsequent care. Some of the barriers may be physical or resource dependent, e.g. the space where the interview takes place or constraints on time. However, there are also nurse–patient barriers – for example, lack of knowledge, embarrassment and fears of being intrusive – that can tend to obscure communication. When considering a patient's intimate sexual behaviours, inevitably the interaction will be influenced by the nurse's own values and beliefs which can sometimes be contrary to the patient's behaviour. Being aware of one's own values, trying to adopt a non-judgemental approach and reflecting on practice may go some way to facilitating communication on sensitive issues such as sex and sexuality, thus providing the patient with better quality care.

This chapter has expressed how important good record-keeping is. The nursing record can be, and has in the past been, used as evidence in courts of law. Records and the information contained within them can either help to promote care or may, if they are incomplete or incorrect, hinder and harm the patient.

It is important that the nurse, midwife and community public health nurse recognize their own limitations and those of the patient. Refer those beyond your capabilities. Recognizing your own prejudices and biases is important when dealing with sensitive and very private information that the patient may or may not choose to give.

CHAPTER THREE

Managing sexual infection

Introduction

STI diagnoses at genitourinary medicine (GUM) clinics have seen an unprecedented rise in the UK. Since 1996 the annual number of diagnoses of gonorrhoea has doubled; with regard to chlamydia there has been an increase of 140 per cent; and syphilis, this once extremely rare infection, has also increased dramatically. It is anticipated that the infection rates are set to rise further (Terence Higgins Trust, 2004). These increases provide health services with a major challenge and nurses can help to confront this challenge.

The most common STIs are chlamydia, non-specific urethritis (NSU) and wart virus. The number of visits to GUM clinics has doubled in the last ten years, with more than a million people visiting GUM clinics (DoH, 2001c). The increasing trend in STIs may in part be related to changes in sexual behaviour (Health Development Agency (HDA), 2004b).

STIs are major causes of public health problems (British Medical Association, 2002) because:

- some STIs have potentially serious outcomes for physical and psychological health;
- some favour and facilitate the spread of HIV infection;
- some may cause serious ill health in mothers and babies;
- some may cause fertility problems.

The WHO (2000) classifies STIs into four groups (see Table 3.1).

This chapter will consider in brief the following STIs:

- gonorrhoea;
- chlamydia;
- syphilis;
- non-specific urethritis;
- *Trichomonas vaginalis*;

Table 3.1 The WHO classification of STIs

Viral infections:

- HIV infection
- Acquired immune deficiency syndrome secondary to HIV infection
- Herpes simplex virus infections
  - Type 1 Herpes simplex virus infection
  - Type 2 Herpes simplex virus infection
- Human papilloma virus infections
- Cytomegalovirus infection
- Hepatitis B infection
- Other sexually transmitted viral infections

Bacterial infections:

- Syphilis
- Gonococci infections
- Chlamydiasis
- Chancroid
- Trichomonal infection
- Gardenerella infections
- Mycoplasma infections
- Other sexually transmitted bacterial infections

Yeast infections:

- Candidiasis
- Other sexually transmitted yeast infections

Infestations:

- Phthirus pubis crab infestation
- Sarcoptes scabiei infestation
- Other sexually transmitted viral infestations

Source: WHO, 2000.

- genital warts;
- genital herpes;
- hepatitis A, B and C;
- HIV.

Making the diagnosis

In order to make a diagnosis the nurse must examine the patient and carry out a range of diagnostic tests. This aspect of the chapter will briefly outline the principles underpinning good practice when examining male and female patients. The tests needed to confirm diagnosis will depend on local policy and procedure and the nurse should refer to the policies and procedures used at a local level. The results of the diagnostic tests have the potential to confirm or eliminate possible infections; it is imperative, therefore, that the nurse carries the tests out with attention to policy and procedure. The following should also be given due consideration:

- the timing of the test(s) (if appropriate);
- the patient is adequately prepared for the test(s);
- the specimens are collected and disseminated efficiently.

One aspect of making a diagnosis is to give the patient the result of the test(s) that have been carried out. The nurse must approach each person as an individual when presenting them with either a positive or negative diagnosis as there may be potential ramifications regarding the test results. Tact and sensitivity are needed and there may be occasions where referral to another agency, e.g. a psychosexual counsellor, is needed as the patient may be experiencing issues of a psychosexual nature.

All patients undergoing intimate examination (and examination of the genitalia is deemed intimate) have the right to have a chaperone present during the examination. The nurse should explain to the patient why the examination is needed and what is to be expected of them, e.g. whether s/he is expected to lie down or stand up prior to undertaking the examination. Time must be given for the patient to ask questions and it is important that informed consent is gained from the patient or the appropriate guardian, in the case of children or those with learning disability.

In order to conduct the examination in a competent and confident manner the nurse will need to understand the function of the male and female genitalia. Important issues such as ensuring privacy, developing a relationship and explaining the procedure have been discussed in Chapter 2.

The Royal College of Obstetricians and Gynaecologists (RCOG) (2002) have produced guidelines concerning intimate examinations. There are no published guidelines specifically related to examination of the male genitalia, despite half of all attendances to genitourinary clinics being male (Rogstad, 2003).

Some nurses may feel uneasy about examining the genitalia and there may be concern if, for example, the patient is male and experiences an erection while the examination is in progress. If the patient does experience an erection the nurse should explain that this is a normal physiological reaction. The examination should continue and the nurse should proceed in a professional and unruffled manner (Bickley, 2002). According to the RCN (2003a) intimate examinations should be conducted in a sensitive and respectful manner.

The examination must be carried out in private, dignity must be protected at all times, and the nurse should help the patient relax. The setting where the examination takes place should be warm and free from interruptions (Collins, 2004). The patient should be assessed holistically and particular attention should be made to respecting any cultural customs or traditions (Dean, 1999). There should be a good light source present in order for the nurse to observe the patient adequately (Estes, 2002). Gloves should be worn whenever there might be contact with body fluids, mucous membranes, or non-intact skin (RCN, 2004b). Epstein et al. (1997) suggest that wearing gloves can emphasize the strictly clinical nature of the examination. Ensure that latex-free gloves are used in order to avoid an allergic reaction to the rubber.

Prior to and during the examination Peate (2005) suggests that the nurse should:

- explain to the patient why the examination is needed and what technique s/he intends to use, e.g. will the patient be expected to stand/sit/lie?
- give the patient an opportunity to ask questions;
- ensure that the patient gives his consent for the examination to take place; local policy may require the nurse to gain written consent prior to the investigation;
- provide information and give explanations in such a manner that the patient understands and has a clear idea of what to expect;
- offer the patient the opportunity to have a chaperone present during the investigation regardless of organizational constraints; if a chaperone cannot be supplied then the nurse must consider, with the patient's agreement, delaying the investigation to a later time in the day or a later date; details of this discussion should be recorded; if the patient refuses an examination this should be documented in the notes;
- not assist the patient in removing clothing unless assistance is required;
- ensure that there are no unnecessary interruptions;
- make certain that the patient's privacy and dignity are protected;
- take into account the wishes of the patient.

The nurse should have the appropriate equipment available in the room before the examination begins in order to avoid having to stop the examination to retrieve additional equipment. The exact type of equipment needed will depend on the purpose of the examination, the site of the infection and the investigation required. French (2004b) suggests the following equipment for the male patient:

- a plastic loop for insertion into the urethra for specimen collection and analysis;

- urine collection apparatus for urinalysis, microscopy, sensitivity and culture;
- dacron tipped throat swab;
- proctoscope for rectal examination and a plastic loop for specimen collection and analysis for those men who report anal sex;
- specific equipment for analysis of prostatic fluid that has been expressed via the urethra following direct prostate massage.

For the female patient:

- a plastic loop for specimens from the posterior fornix of the vagina for specimen collection and analysis;
- a plastic loop to be used for a sample from the endocervix for analysis;
- a plastic loop to obtain a specimen from the proximal urethra for analysis;
- proctoscope for rectal examination and a plastic loop for specimen collection and analysis for those women who report anal sex.

Guidelines have been produced by the Association for Genitourinary Medicine and the Medical Society for the Study of Venereal Diseases (AGUM and MSSVD, 2002) for the management of STIs; these guidelines offer a framework for care provision.

Gonorrhoea

Epidemiology

The number of cases of diagnosed uncomplicated gonorrhoea in 2003 in England, Wales and Northern Ireland stands at 24,157. This is a decrease of 4 per cent compared with 25,065 in 2002. Between 2002 and 2003 the diagnoses fell in men by 4 per cent and women by 3 per cent (HPA, 2004). The highest rates of infection are in young men aged between 20 and 24 years and in women aged between 16 and 19 years of age. Decreased rates have occurred in men aged between 16 and 19 years and women aged between 25 and 34 years of age.

Geographical variations exist with the highest number of diagnoses being made in London for both men and women, 38 per cent and 37 per cent respectively. London also accounted for the highest rates of diagnoses in men which stand at 170 per 100,000 and women 71 per 100,000. Outside of London the West Midlands (68 per 100,000) and the North West of England (64 per 100,000) accounted for the highest rates. Northern Ireland accounted for the lowest rates with an estimated 15 per 100,000 of the population (HPA, 2004).

In Scotland 825 laboratory cases of gonorrhoea were reported in 2003, with the majority of cases occurring in male patients. These men accounted for 81 per cent of the total number (Wallace et al., 2004). Since 2000 the number of episodes has increased by 11 per cent in men and a fall has been noted in women by 37 per cent. Sixty-seven per cent of these cases are among women aged less than 25 years. The increase in male patients is believed to be via men who have sex with men; a doubling of positive rectal specimens has been obtained, raising the diagnoses from 54 to 112 between 2000 and 2003. In Scotland the majority of cases occur within the Greater Glasgow and Lothian NHS Boards; it must be noted that this is where most of Scotland's GUM clinic attendees are situated, and in particular men who have sex with men (HPA, 2004).

The high rates of gonorrhoea appear to be related to geographical variations, with the higher rates being found in urban deprived areas, and also being located within specific population subgroups, such as men who have sex with men (Hughes et al., 2000a). In 2003 22 per cent of all cases of gonorrhoea in men in GUM clinics were acquired through men who have sex with men; 49 per cent of these cases were diagnosed in London.

Causative organism

Gonorrhoea is caused by the gonococcus bacterium and is the clinical disease resulting from infection with the Gram-negative diplococcus *Neisseria gonorrhoeae*. The gonococci are micro-organisms of the species *Neisseria gonorrhoeae* (Robinson, 1998).

Transmission

Transmission occurs with direct inoculation of secretions from one mucous membrane to another. This organism is easily passed on through vaginal, anal and oral sex; close physical contact can also lead to transmission. Vertical transmission can also occur – spreading to mucous membranes such as a baby's eyes. Cross-infection can also occur from the genitals via the fingers to the eyes.

Infection to detection period

The patient may develop symptoms any time between 1 and 14 days.

Clinical manifestations

The clinical manifestations may be systematic or local, uncomplicated or complicated. Robinson (1998) suggests that uncomplicated local infections are seen as urethral infections in men and as urogenital infections in females. The male patient may complain of dysuria, a urethral discharge and epididymitis. There may be pyrexia and tachycardia. The discharge may be noted by the patient as a staining on his underwear. The infection may also be asymptomatic. The female patient may also present with similar signs and symptoms, for example, there may be pyrexia, tachycardia, discharge and abdominal pain. Table 3.2 summarizes the signs and symptoms in males and females.

Table 3.2 The symptoms and signs of gonorrhoea in males and females

Symptoms
Men:

- 80% of cases present with urethral discharge and/or 50% with dysuria
- In less than 10% of cases the infection may be asymptomatic
- Anal discharge occurs in 12% of men who engage in anal intercourse with 7% reporting perianal/anal pain
- 90% of pharyngeal infections are asymptomatic

Women:

- Approximately 50% of women will be asymptomatic
- Vaginal discharge in up to 50% of women is the most common symptom
- 25% of women report lower abdominal pain
- Dysuria but not frequency of micturition is present in 12% of women
- 90% of pharyngeal infections are asymptomatic

Signs
Men:

- A mucopurulent or purulent urethral discharge is common
- Epididymal tenderness and/or swelling and balanitis can occur rarely

Women:

- In 50% of cases a mucopurulent endocervical discharge and easily induced endocervical bleeding can occur
- Less than 5% of women will have pelvic and/or lower abdominal tenderness
- Often when performing an examination no abnormal findings will be noted

Source: Sherrard and Barlow, 1996; Barlow and Philips, 1978; Lewis et al., 1999.

Potential complications

The organism spreads transluminally from the urethra or endocervix to involve the epididymis and prostate gland in less than 1 per cent of males, and the endometrium and pelvic organs in less than 10 per cent of women. Disseminated gonococcal infection is uncommon – less than 1 per cent, disseminating haematologically from infected mucous membranes, resulting in skin lesions, arthralgia, arthritis and tenosynovitis (AGUM and MSSVD, 2002).

Diagnosis

A full sexual history will be needed to assess the patient holistically and arrive at a diagnosis. Diagnosis is confirmed by the presence of *Neisseria gonorrhoeae* at the site of infection. Specimens may be collected from the:

* urethra
* rectum
* oropharynx
* cervix (the cervix is visualized with a speculum) (Daniels, 2002).

Management of care

The patient should be given a full explanation of their condition and particular emphasis should be placed on the potential long-term implications for themselves and their partner. This is best supplemented with clear, accurate, written information. Advice should be given to the patient to refrain from unprotected sexual intercourse until they and their partner(s) have completed treatment and follow up.

Recommended treatment is dependent on each individual patient. The antimicrobial drug of choice is ciprofloxacin 500 mg orally as a single dose or ofloxacin 400 mg as a single dose (Centres for Disease Control and Prevention, 1998). The effective treatment of gonorrhoea has been complicated by the ability of *Neisseria gonorrhoeae* to develop resistance to antimicrobial agents (HPA, 2004). Antimicrobial therapy must take account of local patterns of antimicrobial sensitivity to *Neisseria gonorrhoeae* (FitzGerald and Bedford, 1996).

Special considerations

Neisseria gonorrhoeae may co-exist with other genital mucosal pathogens, for example *Trichomonas vaginalis*, *Candida albicans* and *Chlamydia trachomatis*. Symptoms that the patient presents with may be attributable to co-infecting pathogens. There are several different serotypes or strains (Robinson 1998).

Genital chlamydial infection

Epidemiology

Of all the STIs genital chlamydial infection was the most commonly diagnosed STI in GUM clinics in 2003. The number of uncomplicated chlamydia diagnoses was 82,557 – an 8 per cent increase between 2002 and 2003. As with gonorrhoea the rate of diagnoses has geographical variations.

Of all UK countries England has the highest rates, with rates in London reaching 271 per 100,000. An increase in the number of diagnoses by 10 per cent in men and 7 per cent in women is reported in England, Wales and Northern Ireland. In women the highest rates of diagnoses occur in the 16–19-year age bracket, and for men this is highest in the 20–24 years group (HPA, 2004). In Scotland laboratory diagnoses of genital chlamydia have also continued to rise. In 2003 a reported number of 14,407 is noted compared with 12,392 in 2002, this is a rise of 16 per cent and an 88 per cent rise on recorded diagnoses in 2000 of 7654 (Wallace et al., 2004).

Women suffer the greatest burden of infection. In 1995 diagnoses numbered 17,297; this rose to 49,601 in 2003. Men and women aged less than 25 are at the highest risk of acquiring chlamydia. The HPA (2004) suggest that the increase in the numbers of diagnoses reported may be due to the use of more sensitive laboratory tests.

Causative organism

Chlamydia trachomatis is an obligate intracellular bacterium (Richens, 2004). The common name for *Chlamydia trachomatis* is chlamydia.

Transmission

The key route of transmission is via vaginal intercourse. Chlamydia can also be transmitted via the anus and the orogenital route. Vertical transmission can also occur with pneumonitis and conjunctivitis in the new-born (Conlon and Snydman, 2004; Wakley et al., 2003). Infection sites are the:

- urethra
- cervix
- rectum
- pharynx
- conjunctiva.

Infection to detection period

One to three weeks after exposure.

Clinical manifestations

The number of infections reported is sustained by unrecognized, and therefore untreated, symptoms in both men and women. Table 3.3 outlines the clinical manifestations in men and women. In approximately 80 per cent of women chlamydia is asymptomatic and in men this is 50 per cent. The patient may have pyrexia and tachycardia.

Table 3.3 Clinical features – chlamydial infection

Women:
- Postcoital or intermenstrual bleeding
- Mucopurulent cervicitis, the cervix easily bleeds on contact
- Lower abdominal pain
- Purulent vaginal discharge
- Urethritis
- Pelvic inflammatory disease

Men:
- Urethral discharge
- Dysuria
- Ascending infection leading to epididymitis
- Lower abdominal pain

Men and women:
- Anal discharge, anorectal discomfort
- Proctitis
- Pharyngeal infections, sore throat

Source: Wakley et al., 2003; Robinson, 1998; Richens, 2004.

Potential complications

The bacterium can spread transluminally and lead to pelvic inflammatory disease in women and epididymitis in the male patient. Women may experience infertility and ectopic pregnancy; however, there is little evidence of men experiencing infertility (Wakley et al., 2003). Fitz-Hugh-Curtis syndrome, a liver disorder known as perihepatitis caused by *Chlamydia trachomatis* spreading to the liver, results in inflammation of the capsule of the liver, producing severe and sudden right upper quadrant pain (Peter et al., 2004). The spread of chlamydia may also occur from the fingers to mucous membranes such as the conjunctiva. Wakley et al. (2003) note that, rarely, sexually reactive arthritis known as Reiter's syndrome, an immune-mediated illness, can occur. This results in arthritis, particularly in the ankles and knees, conjunctivitis and uveitis. This is more common in men than women (Conlon and Snydman, 2004).

Diagnosis

A full sexual history will be needed to assess the patient holistically and arrive at a diagnosis. Diagnosing chlamydial infection can be problematic as this is a rapidly developing field (Metters, 1998). The AGUM and the MSSVD (2002) have made recommendations concerning the diagnosis of chlamydia.

In the male patient a first voided urine specimen is as good as, if not better than, a urethral swab (Hay et al., 1991). Patients would prefer to provide a urine specimen as a urethral swab may be painful and uncomfortable. If a urethral swab is to be obtained from the patient then the nurse must gently insert the swab approximately 1–4 cm into the urethra, using a rotating motion once prior to removal. It is recommended that the patient does not void urine for at least one hour (preferably longer) prior to the specimen being given (Chernesky et al., 1997).

A cervical swab is the most effective way of diagnosing chlamydia in the female patient. Hay et al. (1991) would also support the additional use of urethral specimens in assessing infection as 10–20 per cent of additional positive results will be detected in this way. Cervical swabs have high sensitivities – over 80 per cent (Black, 1997). The cervical swab obtained must contain cellular material in order to make a definitive diagnosis. It is suggested (Horner et al., 1998) that more cases may be detected if the specimen is obtained in the later part of the menstrual cycle. The swab should be inserted inside the cervical os and rotated against the endocervix. While a urine specimen is advocated in the male patient, in females this test performs significantly less well than the cervical specimen and as such is not recommended (AGUM and MSSVD, 2002).

Management of care

After the examination has taken place the treatment provided should aim to be effective, easy to take, with a low side effect profile and cause minimum interference with daily lifestyle.

The treatment of uncomplicated chlamydial infection is:

Doxycycline 100 mg orally twice a day for a total of seven days
or
Azithromycin 1 g orally in a single dose.

Weber and Johnson (1995) have demonstrated that the efficacy of antibiotic therapy is questionable but doxycycline and azithromycin have equal efficacy. Azithromycin is considerably more expensive than doxycycline. The clinical decision to use either doxycycline or azithromycin may be based on several factors, not least the patient's lifestyle; azithromycin being best suited to those patients with an erratic lifestyle who may find it difficult to complete a course of therapy (Handsfield and Stamm, 1998).

In order to improve patient concordance with therapy, the nurse should provide the patient with clear written material regarding chlamydia, such as how it is transmitted, the fact that often this is an asymptomatic infection (especially in women), the potential complications if the infection is left untreated, the importance of partner notification, and abstinence from sexual intercourse until after the course of antibiotics has been completed and their partner has been treated (Sanson-Fisher et al., 1992).

Special considerations

All patients who test positive for chlamydial infection should be assessed and screened for other STIs, e.g. gonorrhoea and syphilis. Chlamydial infection may also help in the transmission of HIV, therefore HIV testing should also be considered (Wakley et al., 2003).

Special considerations must be given to pregnant women as doxycycline is contraindicated in pregnancy and the safety of azithromycin in pregnant and lactating women is as yet unspecified (Royal Pharmaceutical Society of Great Britain and British Medical Association, 2004).

New tests for chlamydia are being developed which are carried out on urine samples and from self-administered vulval swabs in women. The Chlamydia Screening Studies (ClaSS) project has been commissioned by the NHS Health Technology Assessment Programme and will consist of six interlinked studies. The National Chlamydia Screening Programme (NCSP) is derived from the National Strategy for Sexual Health (DoH, 2001c). The goal of the NCSP is to control chlamydia through the early detection and treatment of asymptomatic infection; to prevent the development of sequelae; and to reduce onward disease transmission (DoH, 2001c).

Syphilis

Traditionally, acquired syphilis has been classified as either early infectious or late non-infectious; syphilis can also be acquired congenitally. Usually the cut-off point between both of these stages is two years (Adler and French, 2004). Early infectious syphilis can be further divided into primary, secondary or early latent. Tertiary stage syphilis includes gummatous syphilis, cardiovascular and neurological syphilis.

Epidemiology

The HPA (2004) reports that 56 per cent of all diagnoses made between 2002 and 2003 were attributed to men who had sex with men. Large outbreaks of syphilis have been noted in Brighton, Manchester, Newcastle-upon-Tyne, Central Scotland and London. These localized outbreaks of syphilis first occurred in Bristol in 1997 (Doherty et al., 2002). Simms et al. (in press) suggest that there are some factors underlying the change in syphilis epidemiology in the UK that may give some insight into the increase. The outbreak in Bristol was associated with heterosexual intercourse, commercial sex workers, and the use of crack cocaine. The other outbreaks, in Brighton, Manchester, London, Edinburgh and Glasgow, are primarily among men who have sex with men and who may also have a concurrent HIV infection.

The London outbreak is the largest reported to date. Between April 2001 and September 2004 1910 diagnoses were reported. Altogether 1276 diagnoses have been reported in men who have sex with men, 383 in male heterosexuals and the remaining 237 in women (Health Protection Agency, 2004).

In 2003, 1580 new diagnoses of primary and secondary syphilis occurred in England, Wales and Northern Ireland, with an increase of 28 per cent in men and 32 per cent in women. In Scotland during 2003 a total of 67 reports of syphilis were noted, representing an increase of 56 per cent from 43 cases in 2002.

Causative organism

Treponema pallidum, the cause of syphilis, is an anaerobic bacterium (Robinson, 1998). Syphilis is a systemic disease and can lead to a variety of clinical sequelae. After initial inoculation the spirochaete reproduces locally and simultaneously disseminates via the lymphatic system (Conlon and Snydman, 2004).

Transmission

It is only when mucocutaneous syphilitic lesions are present that sexual transmission occurs. Generally transmission occurs via minor abrasions during sexual intercourse; however, transmission can also occur extragenitally.

Vertical transmission may occur from the pregnant women to her foetus as early as the ninth week of gestation (Robinson, 1998).

Infection to detection period

The incubation period can be up to ninety days.

Clinical manifestations

Primary syphilis

At the inoculation site a lesion appears usually within 2–3 weeks (see Table 3.4). This begins as a small papule and ulcerates to become a painless ulcer known as a chancre. Depending on the site of the chancre formation, e.g. the genitals or perineum, localized lymphadenopathy occurs. If left untreated the chancre will heal within 1–2 months.

Table 3.4 Potential sites of primary syphilis

Genital:

• Shaft of penis	• Prepuce
• Coronal sulcus	• Fraenum
• Glans penis	• Urethral meatus
• Fourchette	• Anal margin and canal
• Clitoris	• Rectum
• Vaginal wall	• Labia minora, labia majora
• Cervix	

Extragenital:

• Lip	• Eyelid
• Tongue	• Nipple
• Mouth, tonsil, pharynx	• Any part of the skin or mucous
• Fingers	membranes

Source: Adler and French, 2004.

Secondary syphilis

When dissemination of the spirochaete happens, often within 4–10 weeks after the appearance of the chancre, clinical symptoms will appear. Any organ of the body can be affected; often a rash and lymphadenopathy occur.

Latent syphilis

Secondary syphilis if untreated often resolves spontaneously over several weeks and after this period of time a latent stage occurs where the patient is asymptomatic. Early latent disease occurs within one year of the secondary stage and latent disease, if there have been no symptoms or signs of relapse for over a year.

Tertiary syphilis

After two years or more following the initial infection, late syphilitic symptoms and signs can appear and are characterized as:

- benign late syphilis – gummas, granulomatous lesions of the skin/soft tissue;
- cardiac syphilis – inflammatory aortitis that may lead to an ascending aortic aneurysm, and ischaemic heart disease may be present;
- neurological syphilis – tabes dorsalis and dementia may manifest and there may be episodes of psychosis.

Diagnosis

The patient's history and physical examination can lead the nurse to make a provisional clinical diagnosis; however, it is essential that this is confirmed by laboratory tests (Conlon and Snydman, 2004). *Treponema pallidum* cannot be cultured in vitro and therefore early diagnosis of primary or secondary syphilis depends on dark field microscopy of a specimen taken from a chancre, regional lymph node or other lesion as the treponemes can be detected in the fluid from the chancre. Dark field microscopy is highly sensitive and specific. Examination of the cerebrospinal fluid and X-ray may also be used in the diagnosis (Adler and French, 2004).

Serological testing – for example, Venereal Disease Research Laboratory (VDRL), rapid plasma reagin (RPR) and the Wasserman reaction (WR) – can detect other stages of syphilis. All of these serological tests will detect anticardiolipin antibodies and are 80 per cent positive in cases of primary syphilis and all cases of secondary syphilis (Conlon and Snydman, 2004).

In order to detect antibodies in the patient's serum more specific tests such as fluorescent treponemal antibody absorption test (FTA-Abs) and the *treponemal pallidum* haemagglutination test (TPHA) are available.

Management of care

For over fifty years penicillin has been, and still remains, the drug of choice for the treatment of syphilis. Adler and French (2004) suggest it is the cornerstone of treatment for all types of syphilis. A single injection in the form of benzathine penicillin or a ten-day course of procaine penicillin can be given (Adler and French, 2004). A reaction known as Jarisch-Herxheimer may occur in primary and secondary syphilis and the nurse must warn the patient that fever and flu-like symptoms can occur 3–12 hours after the first injection. In certain instances the chancre or skin lesions can enlarge or become more widespread (Adler and French, 2004). If such a reaction occurs the patient must be reassured and the provision of an antipyretic and a non-steroidal anti-inflammatory drug may help. Table 3.5 provides an overview of the treatment of syphilis.

Table 3.5 A summary of the treatment of syphilis

Stage	Standard treatment	Alternatives
Primary and secondary	Benzathine penicillin 2.4 mega units intramuscularly as a single dose or aqueous procaine penicillin 600 000 units intramuscularly per day for 10 days	Doxycycline 100 mg orally twice per day for 14 days

Table 3.5 continued

Stage	Standard treatment	Alternatives
Latent early (less than two years)	Benzathine penicillin 2.4 mega units intramuscularly as a single dose or aqueous procaine penicillin 600,000 units intramuscularly per day for 10 days	Doxycycline 100 mg orally twice per day for 14 days
Latent late (more than two years)	Aqueous procaine penicillin 900,000 units intramuscularly for 17 days or benzathine penicillin 2.4 mega units intramuscularly weekly over two weeks (three injections)	Doxycycline 100 mg orally twice per day for 30 days
Cardiovascular syphilis	Aqueous procaine penicillin 600,000 units intramuscularly for 17 days (with or without oral prednisolone 20 mg per day starting the day before penicillin treatment and continuing on the same dose for two days after)	Doxycycline 100 mg orally twice per day for 30 days
Gummatous syphilis	Aqueous procaine penicillin 600,000 units intramuscularly for 17 days	Doxycycline 100 mg orally twice per day for 30 days
Neurosyphilis	Aqueous procaine penicillin 2.4 mega units intramuscularly for 17 days (with or without oral prednisolone 20 mg per day starting the day before penicillin treatment and continuing on the same dose for two days after) and oral probenecid 500 mg four times daily	Doxycycline 200 mg orally twice per day for 30 days

Source: Adler and French, 2004.

Special considerations

All patients with syphilis should be screened for other STIs. Penicillin-based regimes are safe to use in pregnancy and breastfeeding (Royal Pharmaceutical Society of Great Britain and British Medical Association, 2004).

Those patients who present with late syphilis should also be tested for HIV as HIV may modify the natural history of syphilis with a more rapid progression to neurosyphilis (Johns et al., 1987).

All patients must be reviewed to ascertain if they have completed treatment; they should also be advised to avoid unprotected sexual intercourse until they and their partner/partners have completed treatment and follow-up. Those patients who have late syphilis will require on-going clinical care and assessment by the most appropriate clinicians.

Non-specific urethritis

Non-specific urethritis (NSU) is inflammation of the urethra and primarily sexually acquired. It is a urethral infection that is not caused by gonorrhoea and is sometimes called non-gonococcal urethritis.

Epidemiology

It is estimated that between 1990 and 1999 approximately 58,528 patients with NSU were seen in GUM clinics in Northern Ireland, Wales and England. The diagnoses of NSU in the UK have remained stable between 1990 and 1999 (Public Health Laboratory Service (PHLS), Department of Health and Social Services and Public Safety (DHSS and PS) and the Scottish Information and Statistics Division (Scottish ISD (D), 2000).

Causative organism

Chlamydia trachomatis is the cause of 30–50 per cent of NSU. The bacteria *Mycoplasma genitalium* and *Ureaplasma urealyticum* are also common causative organisms (Horner et al., 2000; Wakley et al., 2003).

Transmission

This is a condition that is primarily transmitted through sexual intercourse. It may be transmitted by excessive friction when masturbating or an allergic reaction to soap or rubber.

Clinical manifestations

Penile irritation, discharge, dysuria, pyrexia and tachycardia. The condition may also be asymptomatic. Discharge may only be present when the urethra is massaged.

Potential complications

If left untreated NSU may lead to epididymo orchitis and Reiter's syndrome. These complications are rare and occur in less than 1 per cent of cases.

Diagnosis

The presence of a discharge and dysuria may lead to the suspected diagnosis of NSU. However, to confirm diagnosis there must be an excess of polymorphonuclear leucocytes in the anterior aspect of the urethra. A urethral smear is used to obtain the specimen. Mucopurulent cervicitis in the female may also be noted. It must be remembered that NSU may be asymptomatic.

A full explanation of what NSU is should be given to the patient and written information to support verbal advice should be offered. Advice can be offered to explain that sexual intercourse (including masturbation) should cease until after therapy has been completed and the patient's partner/partners have also been treated.

As soon as diagnosis has been made treatment should commence. Antimicrobials have a cure rate of over 95 per cent; they are easy to take, with minimum side effects and the patient can continue with their normal lifestyle with minimum interruption. The treatment suggested for *Chlamydia trachomatis* is as effective for NSU.

Special considerations

All patients who have or who are suspected of having NSU should also have a urethral culture taken for assessment of gonorrhoea and chlamydia. A mid-stream specimen of urine should be obtained and tested (dip stick urinalysis test); if positive for protein and/or glucose, this specimen should be sent for microscopy and culture (Flanagan et al., 1989).

Trichomonas vaginalis

Epidemiology

Data concerning epidemiology of *Trichomonas vaginalis* is scarce. It is suggested that between 1990 and 1999 the diagnoses of *Trichomonas vaginalis* in the UK have doubled in men but remained static in females.

Causative organism

Trichomonas vaginalis is a flagellated protozoon parasite. In women this organism can be found in the vagina, urethra and the paraurethral glands. In men the infection is predominantly located in the urethra (Conlon and Snydman, 2004).

Transmission

In the adult population transmission is exclusively sexually transmitted. *Trichomonas vaginalis* can be transmitted perinatally (Mitchell, 2004) and may occur in 5 per cent of babies born to infected mothers (Robinson and Ridgway, 1994).

Infection to detection period

Usually seven days with a range of 3–21 days.

Clinical manifestations

Between 10 and 50 per cent of cases in females are asymptomatic and in men this is between 15 and 50 per cent. Usually men present as sexual partners of infected women (Fouts and Kraus, 1980).

Table 3.6 outlines the symptoms and signs associated with *Trichomonas vaginalis*.

Table 3.6 An outline of symptoms and signs of *Trichomonas vaginalis*

Symptoms
Men:
- Urethral discharge is the commonest symptom and this may occur with or without dysuria
- Urethral irritation
- Frequency of micturition
- Rarely prostatitis

Women:
- Vaginal discharge
- Vulval itching
- Dysuria
- Malodorous urine
- There may be low abdominal discomfort

Signs
Men:
- Small to moderate amounts of urethral discharge

- Asymptomatic
- Rarely balanoposthitis

Women:
- Vaginal discharge, varying in consistency from thin and scanty to profuse and thick
- Discharge may be frothy and yellow
- Vulvitis and vaginitis
- Strawberry coloured cervix seen on colposcopic examination
- Asymptomatic

Source: adapted from AGUM and MSSVD, 2002.

Potential complications

There is evidence to suggest that *Trichomonas vaginalis* may have a detrimental effect on a pregnancy outcome and can also be associated with pre-term delivery and low birth weight (Cotch et al., 1997; Saurina and McCormack, 1997). Sorvillo and Kerndt (1998) have suggested that there may be evidence indicating that *Trichomonas vaginalis* enhances HIV transmission.

Diagnosis

An examination of the external genitalia may appear normal in both sexes. In the female the vaginal and vulval wall may demonstrate erythema (Mitchell, 2004). In the male patient a urethral swab is required, combined with a urine sample to confirm diagnosis. A swab is taken from the top of the vagina in women; urine specimens in the female patient are less reliable (Wakley et al., 2003). Mitchell (2004) concludes that diagnosis should be made by direct microscopy of discharge and urine (in the male). Microscopy can reveal the flagellated organism and there will be increased numbers of polymorphs (Conlon and Snydman, 2004).

Management of care

Both sexual partner(s) should be treated and sexual abstinence is advised until treatment is completed (Mitchell, 2004). Screening for coexistent STIs is advised in both the man and the woman.

   Trichomonas vaginalis is susceptible to metronidazole (or tinidazole – a related drug) with an associated 95 per cent cure rate (Conlon and Snydman, 2004; Mitchell, 2004). Metronidazole 2 g orally in a single dose or metronidazole 400 to 500 mg twice daily for 5–7 days is recommended. Approximately 20–25 per cent of cases are cured spontaneously (Forna and Gulmezoglu, 2000).

Special considerations

Metronidazole is contraindicated in the first trimester of pregnancy and safety in pregnancy has not as yet been determined. High single dose regimens during pregnancy should be avoided (Royal Pharmaceutical Society of Great Britain and British Medical Association, 2004).

The nurse should advise the patient not to use alcohol while taking metronidazole as a disulfiram type of reaction may occur. Disulfiram – an anti-alcoholic medication – produces a sensitivity to alcohol which can result in an unpleasant reaction, even if small amounts of alcohol have been taken.

Genital warts (anogenital warts)

Genital warts are often referred to as anogenital warts or condylomata acuminata. Genital warts are the clinically visible manifestations of infection with human papillomavirus (HPV) and in England, Wales and Northern Ireland they are the most prevalent diagnosed STI.

Epidemiology

The diagnoses of genital warts increased by 2 per cent between 2002 and 2003. The number of diagnoses increased in 2003 to 70,665 from 65,569 cases in 2002. Fifty-three per cent of diagnoses were in men and 47 per cent associated were in women in 2003. In men aged 20–24 years the number of diagnoses was highest, for women the age group was 16 to 24 years. The greatest proportional increase in numbers of new episodes of genital warts was seen in men aged under 16 years and in women this was in the over 40 years age group (HPA, 2004).

Geographically, London has the highest rates; outside of London this was followed by the North West and North East of England. In the South East of England, however, there has been a decrease of 6 per cent. In Northern Ireland and Wales the rates have also decreased. In Scotland data suggest that there are fewer than 119 diagnoses per 100,000 of the population (HPA, 2004).

Causative organism

The virus human papillomavirus (HPV) is the causative organism that results in warts; there have been over 90 genotypes identified. Genital warts are associated with genotype 6 and 11; phenotypes 16, 18, 31 and 45 are associated with the development of invasive cervical carcinoma and certain cancers of the anogenital tract (International Agency for Research on Cancer, 1996; Conlon and Snydman, 2004).

Transmission

The mode of transmission is primarily sexual; however, HPV may be transmitted perinatally and from digital lesions – no evidence is available to suggest that transmission is possible via foamites.

Clinical manifestations

The most common clinical presentation is papules in the anogenital region. Genital warts often result in little physical discomfort; however, they are disfiguring and can result in psychological distress (Clarke et al., 1996). Irritation and soreness can occur particularly in the anal region. If urinary flow becomes obstructed or distorted and there is haematuria or rectal bleeding, this may suggest internal lesions.

Table 3.7 outlines the signs associated with genital warts.

Table 3.7 Signs of genital warts

- Lesions are most common at the site of trauma in sexual intercourse but lesions can occur at other sites
- In both sexes peri-anal lesions can and do occur; however, these are seen more often in homosexual men
- Occult lesions may be seen in the following:
  - The vagina
  - The cervix
  - Urethral meatus
  - Anal canal
- Extra-genital lesions can occur in the following:
  - Oral cavity
  - Larynx
  - Conjunctivae
  - Nasal cavity

Source: adapted from Sonnex et al., 1991; Rymark et al., 1993.

Diagnosis

Diagnosis is made on the clinical appearance of the warts as HPV cannot be cultured. If there is any doubt concerning the nature of the lesions, for example if they appear atypical or pigmented, then a biopsy is required prior to therapeutic intervention.

Management of care

The patient should be given a full explanation of the condition, and time should be spent (supplemented by written information) explaining the potential long-term complications for their health and the health of their partner.

The use of condoms may prevent the transmission of HPV to an uninfected partner(s); some patients may prefer to use a condom while the warts are visible. The psychological impact of warts is for some patients the worst aspect of the condition; the nurse needs to spend time listening to and attempting to alleviate any psychological distress that the patient may encounter. Referral for counselling may be appropriate.

There are several types of treatment available and some are more effective than others. The mode of treatment should be discussed with the patient, taking into account their lifestyle.

Topical chemicals such as podophyllin, podophylotoxin and trichloroacetic acid are ineffective, especially when the lesion occurs on keratinized skin (Conlon and Snydham, 2004). Soft non-keratinized warts do respond well to podophyllin, podophylotoxin and trichloroacetic acid.

Keratinized lesions are treated more effectively with physical ablative therapy such as cryotherapy, excision or electrocautery; cervical lesions may be treated with laser therapy. Surgical excision may be required for extensive lesions (Conlon and Snydham, 2004).

Special considerations

It has been noted that there is a relationship between invasive cervical cancer and other cancers of the anogenital tract; the patient must be made aware of this and a referral to the appropriate health care professional may be needed. As genital warts are often sexually transmitted, the patient should be asked if they would agree to further investigations to rule out any other STIs.

Genital herpes

Epidemiology

The HPA (2004) report that there have been 17,932 diagnoses of genital herpes simplex made in GUM clinics in Northern Ireland, England and Wales; in Scotland 1310 laboratory reports of infection with genital herpes simplex have been reported in 2003. There has been an overall increase of 3 per cent between 2002 and 2003. Excluding Scotland, the number of diagnoses decreased by 2 per cent in men and 3 per cent in women; the female to male ratio remains stable at 1.7:1. Diagnostic rates were highest among those aged between 20 and 24 years of age. For the first time since 1998 rates of diagnosed genital herpes have fallen; time will tell if this is an ongoing trend in rates of diagnosis.

Across the UK rates appear to be evenly distributed, lowest rates being observed in Northern Ireland, North East England and Wales. London has the highest rates, with twenty-eight per cent of all diagnoses (HPA, 2004).

Causative organism

The herpes simplex virus types I and II (HSV I+II) are responsible for causing genital herpes. Type I is predominantly responsible for causing infections that are seen on the face and type II for the infections associated with the genitalia (Wakley et al., 2003). Brugha et al. (1997) have noted that there are increasing numbers of genital herpes infections that are caused by HSV I.

Transmission

Transmission occurs almost exclusively via skin to skin contact.

Infection to detection period

The average incubation period from infection to symptoms is 3–7 days (Conlon and Snydman, 2004).

Clinical manifestations

Fifty per cent of those with primary infections are asymptomatic. Primary infection results in latent infection of the sacral root ganglia, with the possibility of subsequent periodical reactivation and this may be asymptomatic or symptomatic.

Table 3.8 provides details of the signs and symptoms associated with genital herpes.

Table 3.8 Signs and symptoms of genital herpes

- Asymptomatic
- Tingling itching and burning sensation
- Myalgia
- Pyrexia
- Malaise
- Painful ulceration
- Dysuria
- Vaginal/urethral discharge
- Blistering ulceration of the genitalia: the external genitalia are the most frequently involved; however, lesions may be confined to the cervix or to the rectum
- Inguinal lymphadenopathy

Source: Cowan, 2004; Conlon and Snydman, 2004.

Potential complications

Autonomic neuropathy that may result in urinary retention and aseptic meningitis (AGUM and MSSVD, 2001) is a potential complication. If neonatal transmission occurs, this carries with it a high mortality rate and may lead to damage to the brain, skin and eyes.

Diagnosis

Diagnosis is often made on clinical appearance and there are typical vesicles and ulcers. However, Cowan (2004) suggests that diagnosis based on observation alone is suboptimal; diagnosis must be confirmed by culture.

Electron microscopy can also be used to confirm diagnosis. Serological tests will be able to determine if the infection is due to HSV I or HSV II (Conlon and Snydman, 2004). Isolation of the virus is made by taking a specimen from the lesion directly by culture, polymerase chain reaction or antigen detection (Cowan, 2004). The specimen taken from the lesion should be taken from the base of the ulcer and it is vital that rapid transporting of the specimen is achieved.

Management of care

The nurse should provide the patient with analgesia and it can be helpful to encourage the patient to engage in regular baths to ease the pain. There is a range of oral anti-viral drugs available:

- aciclovir
- valaciclovir
- famciclovir.

These drugs are highly effective in reducing severity and duration of the infection; oral medications are more effective than topical agents. The medication should be commenced as soon as possible after the symptoms occur, even if the symptoms and signs seem to be mild. It is recommended that treatment be commenced as this may prevent more severe symptoms developing (Cowan, 2004). If the patient is vomiting and cannot tolerate the oral preparation then intravenous therapy may need to be considered.

Table 3.9 provides the recommended drug regimens.

Table 3.9 Drug recommendations for genital herpes

- Aciclovir 200 mg five times daily for five days
- Famciclovir 250 mg three times a day for five days
- Valaciclovir 500 mg twice daily for five days

Source: AGUM and MSSVD, 2001.

It is important that the patient knows that the infection cannot be eradicated, merely managed. Since this is the case some patients may need to be provided with support to come to terms with this sometimes severe and stigmatizing diagnosis. R. Patel et al. (1999) consider the quality of life of patients who have genital herpes. Cowan (2004) states that the provision of appropriate psychological support and the correct information may prevent the development of severe psychological sequelae.

Special considerations

The patient may require hospitalization if there is urinary retention and/or meningism. The management of women in pregnancy and during labour is complex and the reader should consult local policy; Hensleigh et al. (1996) discuss these important issues further.

The hepatitides A, B and C

Epidemiology

Notifications of hepatitis A (HAV) have increased; in 1998, 1515 cases had been notified and this had risen to 1676 in 1999. HAV is common worldwide. Hepatitis B (HBV) has also increased from 886 cases in 1998 and 864 in 1999 to 1035 in 2000. There has been an ongoing increase in the numbers of cases of hepatitis C (HCV): 5745 cases had been notified in 1999 in comparison with 4483 in 1998. HBV is estimated to affect 300 million people worldwide and approximately 0.3 per cent of the UK population. HCV estimations worldwide are approximately 170 million; in the UK this is estimated as 0.4 per cent of the population (DoH, 2002b). See Table 3.10 for a comparison of the hepatitides A to C.

Table 3.10 A comparison of the hepatitides A to C

Hepatitis type	Diagnosis	Incubation period	Transmission routes
A	Serology	2 to 6 weeks	Faeco-oral
B	Serology	8 to 12 weeks (maybe up to 24 weeks)	Parenteral, perinatal or sexual
C	Serology	4 to 8 weeks (maybe up to 24 weeks)	Parenteral, perinatal or sexual

Source: Gilson, 2004.

Hepatitis A

Causative organism

HAV is a ribonucleic acid picorna virus. It is common in parts of the world where sanitation is poor and predominantly affects children.

Transmission

The route for transmission is via the faeco-oral route, hence its predominance in children. Those patients who engage in oro-anal sex are also at risk of transmitting the virus.

Clinical manifestations

Approximately 50 per cent of patients may be asymptomatic.
   The prodromal phase includes:

- malaise
- myalgia
- fatigue.

There may be upper right abdominal pain and jaundice can occur with:

- anorexia
- fatigue
- nausea
- itching
- steatorrhoea
- dark urine
- hepatomegaly
- dehydration.

Potential complications

In 0.4 per cent of cases fulminant hepatitis occurs; however, some 15 per cent of cases will require hospitalization with severe hepatitis (Fagan and Williams, 1990). There is an association with an increased rate of miscarriage and premature labour as a result of the infection (Medhat et al., 1993).

Management of care

All patients should be advised to refrain from food handling and unprotected sexual intercourse until they have become non-infectious. The patient needs an explanation about the infection and the potential harm it can cause themselves and others.

The patient should be prevented from becoming dehydrated and will need advice about how to maintain hydration. Prescribed anti-histamines may help but caution must be taken if liver function has been compromised.

Special considerations

HAV is a notifiable infection. A vaccine is available that can be given for single immunization for HAV or conjointly with immunization against HAV and HBV. The nurse should provide health education in order to stress the routes of transmission and ways in which this can be reduced.

Hepatitis B

Causative organism

This virus is a deoxyribonucleic acid virus, a hepadna virus. HBV is endemic worldwide with high carriage rates noted in particular parts of the world.

Transmission

Transmission can occur sexually with homosexual men, heterosexuals and sex workers (Gilson, 2004). Transmission is via blood, blood products, drug users who share drug injecting paraphernalia, needle stick injury, use of acupuncture needles and vertically from mother to child (Conlon and Snydman, 2004).

Clinical manifestations

Asymptomatic infection is found in approximately 10–50 per cent of adults in the acute phase. The prodromal phase can reflect the signs and symptoms noted in HAV; however, with HBV these can be much more severe and prolonged (McIntyre, 1990). After many years of infection and in relation to duration and severity, Hoofnagle (1990) notes that there may be signs of chronic liver disease:

- spider naevi
- finger clubbing
- jaundice
- hepato-splenomegaly
- ascites
- haematoma formation
- encephalopathy

Potential complications

The potential complications are as with HAV, but the increased morbidity associated with HBV should be noted. Ten per cent of patients who develop cirrhosis of the liver will progress to liver cancer (Hoofnagle, 1990). Symptoms are exacerbated where the patient has liver disease and uses high levels of alcohol.

Management of care

Initially management will be the same as for HAV.

Interferon alpha has been used in the treatment of HBV with some success and further trials are being conducted into the possibility of using new antiviral treatments (BMA, 2002). The reader is advised to consult more definitive texts outlining the treatment of HBV; treatment options are varied and will depend on a variety of factors.

Special considerations

As for HAV. The patient should be advised not to donate blood, semen, tissue or organs (Alter, 1997). HBV is a notifiable disease.

Hepatitis C

Causative organism

Hepatitis C (HCV) is a ribonucleic acid virus of the flavivridae group. This virus is also endemic worldwide with particular areas of the world having high prevalence rates, for example, East Asia and Eastern Europe (Alter, 1997).

Transmission

The majority of cases are via the parenteral route:

- intravenous drug users;
- transfusion of blood/blood products;
- renal dialysis;
- needle stick injury;
- sharing a razor with an HCV positive individual;
- sexual transmission (very low rates);
- vertical transmission (very low rates).

Clinical manifestations

Over 80 per cent of patients are asymptomatic. Early stages are similar to both HAV and HBV.

Potential complications

It has been noted that between 50 and 80 per cent of infected patients will become chronic carriers of HCV; they may also be asymptomatic (Bonkovsky and Wooley, 1999). Complications associated with pregnancy are the same as for HAV.

Management of care

Initially the management of care will be the same as for HAV.

Treatment of HCV with interferon alpha combined with ribavirin has been shown to be effective in 25–40 per cent of cases (BMA, 2002). The reader is advised to consult more definitive texts outlining the treatment of HCV; treatment options are varied and will depend on a variety of factors.

Special considerations

As for HAV/HBV. HCV is a notifiable disease.

Human immunodeficiency virus

The human immunodeficiency virus (HIV) was first detected in 1983 (Williams and Weller, 2004). The rise in the numbers of cases of HIV since 1998 continues. This section of the chapter gives only a brief overview of the issues associated with HIV and the reader is advised to consult other texts/literature to develop a deeper understanding of the key issues associated with HIV.

Epidemiology

The annual total of 6606 diagnoses, as reported by the end of June 2004, was more than double the number of diagnoses in 1998; at that time the number stood at 2835 (HPA, 2004). Effective use of highly active anti-retroviral therapy (HAART) was introduced in the mid-1990s, and the use of such therapies has meant that there has been a decline in the number of AIDS diagnoses and deaths in HIV infected people.

The number of diagnoses in heterosexuals has increased and since 1999 the number of new HIV diagnoses in the heterosexual population has exceeded the number of diagnoses among men who have sex with men. Men who have sex with men, however, remain the group at highest risk of acquiring HIV in the UK. Table 3.11 considers the exposure category of

HIV infections that have been diagnosed in the UK to the end of 2003 since 1999.

Table 3.11 Exposure category of HIV infections in the UK: to the end of 2003

Year of diagnosis	Men who have sex with men	Heterosexual men and women	Injecting drug use	Mother to infant	Blood/ blood products	Other/ undeter- mined[2]	Total (100%)
1999	1367 (44%)	1437 (47%)	112 (4%)	78 (3%)	21 (0.7%)	73 (2%)	3088
2000	1516 (39%)	2007 (52%)	112 (3%)	103 (3%)	24 (1%)	90 (2%)	3852
2001	1765 (35%)	2878 (57%)	134 (3%)	94 (2%)	25 (0%)	114 (3%)	5040
2002[1]	1809 (30%)	3566 (59%)	106 (2%)	106 (2%)	30 (0%)	400 (7%)	6071
2003[1]	1735 (26%)	3801 (58%)	107 (2%)	133 (2%)	28 (0%)	802 (12%)	6606

(1) Numbers will rise as further reports are received. (2) The proportion with exposure category undetermined is always higher for the most recent year because of the time needed to complete follow-up. Source: HPA, 2004.

Causative organism

HIV is the causative organism and is a member of the retrovirus family. HIV type I infects T lymphocytes (CD4+ cells), semen and other tissues and cells throughout the body including (Conlon and Snydman, 2004):

- plasma cells
- macrophages
- brain.

With an outbreak of viral replication there is a decline in the CD4+ T lymphocytes and this results in decreased cellular immunity. The level of CD4+ cells and the T lymphocyte count are strongly correlated with the association between the risks of developing opportunistic infections.

Transmission

HIV is transmitted by:

- sexual contact;
- blood to blood contact (i.e. needlestick injury);
- vertical transmission.

Infection to detection period

Conlon and Snydman (2004) suggest that once a patient is infected it may take weeks or months to develop detectable antibodies to HIV. Seroconversion takes approximately 45 days.

Clinical manifestations

In some instances a patient may remain asymptomatic for at least a year (Pratt, 2003). People with HIV can and do look and feel healthy; most of the time, the virus damages the immune system slowly and the patient gradually becomes less able to defend him/herself from infection and recover from these infections. The patient becomes infected with particular types of cancer and infections (opportunistic infections) that would not normally affect a person with an intact immune system. Table 3.12 describes some of the common clinical manifestations associated with primary HIV infection.

Table 3.12 Some of the common clinical manifestations associated with primary HIV infection

Fever (> 38°C)
Fatigue
Erythematous maculopapular rash
Myalgia
Headache
Pharyngitis
Cervical lymphadenopathy
Arthralgia
Oral ulcers
Odynaphagia
Axillary lymphadenopathy
Weight loss
Nausea
Diarrhoea
Night sweats
Cough
Inguinal lymphadenopathy
Abdominal pain
Oral candidiasis
Vomiting
Photophobia
Sore eyes
Genital ulcers
Tonsillitis
Depression
Dizziness

Source: Hawkins, 2002.

Potential complications

Potentially, HIV is a life-threatening disease and an immune system that is not fully intact can lead to the development of opportunist infections and HIV associated malignancies. Almost 50 per cent of people with HIV will eventually develop AIDS if they are not treated (BMA, 2002).

Diagnosis

Seroconversion is determined by the presence of serum antibodies to HIV on enzyme immunoassay followed by confirmation testing using Western blotting techniques (Conlon and Snydman, 2004). When serological results are unclear then HIV DNA or RNA polymerase chain reaction may be used in order to confirm infection (Pratt, 2003).

Management of care

At this moment in time there is no cure for HIV infection nor is there any vaccine that can protect against it (DoH, 2002b). The management and care of people infected with HIV is no different than the care provided to any other patient who may have a chronic condition with multiple pathology. People with HIV require skilled care provided by a confident and competent practitioner. Understanding the pathophysiology associated with the disease can help to equip the nurse with the confidence and competence required. Often stigma and misunderstanding can complicate issues; above all the nurse must provide care that is based on individual needs and in a non-judgemental manner, adhering to the tenets of the NMC (2004a).

Modern combination treatment HAART, consisting of taking three or more drugs, has transformed HIV from a fatal illness to a treatable chronic condition. Some 25 per cent of new HIV cases may be resistant to one or more of the antiviral therapies used in the treatment; resistance may also occur and treatment can become suboptimal if concordance to treatment regimens is not maintained (BMA, 2002).

Special considerations

The timing of the HIV test is important; it may take weeks or months for antibodies to HIV to appear in the blood. If a patient requests a test soon after exposure to HIV, antibodies may not have developed; this is known as the window period. The result of the test at this stage may be inaccurate and the patient may receive a false negative result. Wakley et al. (2003) suggest that the patient is re-tested after three months in order to obtain a definitive result.

There are particular implications for having an HIV test and the patient needs to be aware of these prior to having a test – whether or not the patient has tested positive or negative to HIV – for example:

- life insurance may become expensive;
- it may be difficult to obtain a loan;
- problems may occur with mortgages that are backed by life insurance;
- travel to certain parts of the world is prohibited if the patient is HIV positive;
- immigration to some countries may be thwarted if the patient is HIV positive;
- there may be implications for their occupation, e.g. if they are a health care worker their practice may need to be changed.

Conclusion

In order to care for patients and their partner(s) with STIs the nurse needs to have an in-depth understanding of the range of conditions with which they may come into contact. Understanding the fundamental facts about the various STIs and how they may be transmitted are the first steps towards preventing them. There may be short- and long-term effects associated with a variety of STIs.

While it is healthy for people to enjoy active sex lives, it must also be noted that there are over 25 STIs, some of which if left untreated may lead to serious short- and long-term harm. This chapter has provided the reader with a brief outline of nine STIs; a framework has been provided for the nurse to address individual patient needs. The reader is advised to develop and build upon current knowledge in order to provide care that is based on best available evidence as opposed to ritual, hearsay and tradition.

Table 3.13 summarizes the nine STIs discussed in this chapter.

Table 3.13 A summary of the nine STIs discussed in this chapter

Infection	Characteristics	Comments
Gonorrhoea	Can be asymptomatic Men: purulent penile discharge, dysuria, frequency of micturition Women: dysuria, altered vaginal discharge, abnormal menses	Rectal infection Pharyngeal infection

Table 3.13 continued

Infection	Characteristics	Comments
Syphilis	Primary: chancre – may be multiple, painful, purulent Secondary: multi-systemic infection, rash (soles and feet), mucocutaneous lesions, generalized lymphadenopathy Tertiary: cardiac, neurologic, ophthalmic, auditory, gummatous lesions	Three stages: early, late and tertiary. Can be congenital
Chlamydia	Can be asymptomatic Men: Urethral discharge, dysuria Women: Postcoital or intermenstrual bleeding, mucopurulent cervicitis	The most prevalent STI to date May be rectal symptoms – anal discharge, proctitis Pharyngeal infection
Non-specific urethritis	Can be asymptomatic Urethral discharge, dysuria, penile irritation	Predominantly caused by *Chlamydia trichomatis* Can result in reactive arthritis, Reiter's syndrome
Trichomonas	Male: often asymptomatic Women: malodorous vaginal discharge, thin, foamy discharge (yellow/green) causes itching of the vulva and vagina, dysuria, dyspareunia. Lower abdominal discomfort	Almost exclusively sexually transmitted
Genital herpes	No typical presentation, generally: Tingling, burning, itching sensations, blistering and ulceration in the genital and/or perianal areas Urethral discharge, vaginal discharge, dysuria Pyrexia, myalgia	Caused by herpes simplex virus type 1 and 2 Can have a profound psychological impact
Genital warts	Single or multiple spots, may be painless, can cause itching, soft or keratinized, broad based or pimple	Caused by the human papilloma virus, 20 types detected Types 6 and 11 most common form of visible warts Types 16, 18, 31, 33 and 35 associated with cervical dysplasia Can have a profound psychological impact

Table 3.13 continued

Infection	Characteristics	Comments
HIV	A multi-system disease related to a depleted immune system Fatigue, diarrhoea, weight loss, generalized persistent lymphadenopathy, anorexia, night sweats	Increasing heterosexual transmission. Men who have sex with men still the group at greatest risk of acquiring HIV
Hepatitides	Hepatitis A, B, C Can be asymptomatic Hepatitis A: commonly transmitted via the oro-faecal route or by contaminated food Hepatitis B: sexual transmission is the main route, parenteral and vertical transmission noted Hepatitis C: transmitted via parenteral route, blood and blood products	As yet no immunization available Can have a profound psychological impact Immunizations against hepatitis A and B Currently no immunization available for hepatitis C

CHAPTER FOUR

Sexual health counselling: using counselling skills

Introduction

The Oxford English Dictionary defines counselling as 'to advise, to give advice to people professionally on social problems'. Nurses support and give advice to patients in a variety of ways in their everyday work. However, nurses are not counsellors and it would not be possible in a chapter of this size to provide the nurse with a comprehensive counselling guide.

The nurse should aim to provide the patient with an opportunity to offer his/her support, allow the patient to refuse that support, and when appropriate give an opportunity to work through complex issues relating to sexual health needs. Provision of information is paramount; it is equally important that the nurse allows the patient to explore these issues from a practical and emotional perspective. This chapter addresses some of the issues the nurse may find him/herself dealing with when working with patients within the field of sexually transmitted infections. It also provides an insight into the complex issues associated with information, advice and support provision.

Key terms

Some people are counsellors offering advice to others in a professional context, for example financial counsellors; others undertake training in order to call themselves counsellors and this can vary from a few weeks to a number of years and indeed, for some, this training may never end. The overall aim of counselling according to the British Association for Counselling (1996) is:

> to provide an opportunity for the client to work towards living in a more resourceful way ... Counselling may be concerned with developmental issues, addressing and resolving specific problems, making decisions, coping with crisis, developing personal insights and knowledge, working through feelings

of inner conflict or improving relationships with others. The counsellor's role is to facilitate the client's work in ways which respect the client's values, personal resources and capacity for self determination [3.1] [...] Counselling involves a deliberately undertaken contract with clearly agreed boundaries and commitment to privacy and confidentiality. It requires explicit and informed agreement [3.2].

When considering the above statement there are many implications for any nurse and particularly the nurse who offers help and advice to patients who are or who have been affected by an STI. The DoH (2001f) defines counselling as:

a systematic process which gives individuals an opportunity to explore, discover and clarify ways of living more resourcefully, with a greater sense of well being. Counselling may be concerned with addressing and resolving specific problems, making decisions, coping with crises, working through conflict, or improving relationships with others.

Figure 4.1 conceptualizes the nature of counselling.

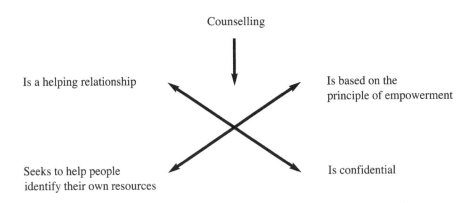

Figure 4.1 A conceptual view of the nature of counselling. Source: Hough, 2003.

Russell (2002) suggests that the nurse may conclude that he/she is involved in counselling; however, he states that this only becomes a counselling relationship when the recipient agrees to enter into such a relationship, anything else in this context would be the use of counselling skills. Burnard (1995) advises that using counselling skills is not the same as counselling. There are indeed similar features, but they are different; as the British Association for Counselling (1996) state, it is the kind of relationship that is the determining factor. In order to avoid confusion, Russell

(2002) prefers to use the term therapeutic communication. It should be noted that there are close relationships between:

- counselling;
- communication skills;
- counselling skills.

Freshwater (2002) considers the use of the term therapeutic nursing and draws on the work of Muetzel (1988) who describes the activities and factors affecting the therapeutic nurse–patient relationship. Muetzel (1988) contends that for the nurse to develop and enhance the therapeutic relationship then s/he must develop as a person, both personally and professionally. Clark et al. (1991) use a hierarchical approach to demonstrate the three relationships stated above. There are associations and links with training, and increased self-awareness for both the client and practitioner. When the nurse uses counselling skills appropriately they provide the patient with opportunities to become more self-aware, and in so doing Sully (2003) suggests that the patient has the ability to make more informed choices. Being able to make more informed choices empowers the patient in any situation, including making informed choices for example about treatment and safer sex activities within the realm of sexual health. Table 4.1 describes the hierarchical relationships between communication skills, counselling and counselling skills.

Table 4.1 An overview of counselling, counselling skills and communication skills

Counselling
The purpose is to:
Offer time, respect and attention to help a person find ways, resourcefully

The skills required to do this are:
Being able to build a trusting, confidential relationship over time and receive supervision

Counselling skills
The purpose is to:
Facilitate greater awareness and understanding of a problem, to help clients help themselves

The skills required to do this are:
- Being self-aware
- Being empathic
- Providing genuineness
- Being accepting
- Providing reflective listening
- Paraphrasing
- Clarifying

Table 4.1 continued

- Helping to set achievable goals/objectives
- Enabling and facilitating catharsis
- Appropriate self-disclosure

Communication skills
The purpose is to:
- Provide information
- Allow discussion and dialogue
- Allow expression of feelings
- Support and educate
- Assess a situation

The skills required to do this are:
- Observing
- Listening
- Asking open-ended questions
- Being aware of body language
- Using silence and touch
- Being able to identify and make appropriate referrals

Source: adapted from Clark et al., 1991.

O. Slevin (2003) offers another approach to differentiating the various ranges of counselling activities. He suggests that there is an assortment of counselling activities, from guidance – a highly directive and structured approach – to counselling where the approach could be said to be non-directive and unstructured (see Table 4.2).

Table 4.2 The range of activities associated with counselling

Guidance	Advice	Counselling
• Highly directive • Highly structured • The counsellor determines; the client accepts • Closed: addresses specific issues • Information content high • Demands competence in communication skills	• Moderately directive • Semi-structured • The counsellor determines with the client's agreement • Flexible: issues broadly agreed • Information content moderate • Demands competence in interpersonal skills	• Highly non-directive • Mainly unstructured • The client determines; the counsellor facilitates • Open: addresses emerging issues • Information content low • Demands competence in relational skills
Counsellor is a guide	Counsellor is an advisor	Counsellor is a therapist

Source: O. Slevin, 2003.

The contribution nurses make in advising and helping patients must never be underestimated. Burnard (1999) suggests that all nurses should be taught counselling skills to enable them to help and support patients with their problems in a positive therapeutic manner. By using counselling skills the nurse can help the patient to have more of an awareness of their strengths and weaknesses and, by becoming more aware, this may help the patient to help themselves. Table 4.3 outlines some of the counselling skills that have been suggested by Burnard (1999).

Table 4.3 Some suggested counselling skills for nurses

- Listening and attending: listening without being judgemental, giving the person your full attention
- Using open-ended questions: try to use questions that begin with 'how', 'what', 'where' and 'when', enabling the person to expand on their response
- Reflecting: reflecting thoughts – echoing the last few words that the person has used, reflecting feelings – echoing the feelings or unstated thoughts which underline a statement. Caution should be used with this technique so as not to overuse it.
- Summarizing: pulling together all of the different strands that the person has brought with them during the conversation and as a result of this help the person to organize their thoughts. Bring to an end the therapeutic conversation
- Seeking clarification: checking for understanding by asking the person

Source: adapted from Burnard, 1999.

Using counselling skills to provide help to patients can occur in various clinical situations, for example:

- pre- and post-HIV testing;
- sexuality issues;
- when providing the result of a diagnosis, e.g. genital warts;
- when discussing relationships, e.g. when deciding on patient notification;
- caring for those affected by rape and/or sexual abuse.

Choice of counselling interventions available

Just as there is a range and a great diversity among patients and nurses, there is also a range of counselling interventions that are available. The choice of intervention is very much dependent upon the skill of the nurse, the patient and the context of care. It is estimated that there are at least 300–400 models of counselling and psychotherapy available. The DoH (2001f) has produced evidence-based clinical practice guidelines related to treatment choice in psychological therapies and counselling; these guidelines have the potential to influence the choice of intervention. The guidelines provide an evidence base that will help to determine who is likely to benefit from psychological treatment, and what therapies are most suitable for which patient. The scope of the guidelines is relevant to the following problems that the patient with a sexually transmitted infection may present with:

- depression, including suicidal behaviour;
- anxiety, panic disorder, social anxiety and phobias;
- post-traumatic disorders;
- obsessive compulsive disorders;
- personality disorders, including repetitive self-harm.

Counselling intervention can take place in a variety of environments and contexts (both statutory and non-statutory provision) (see Table 4.4).

Table 4.4 Examples of venues and contexts in which counselling may occur

- One to one
- With and within groups
- With couples (partners)
- Face to face
- Over the telephone
- Electronically, e.g. via email, Internet
- Outreach
- Hospital based, e.g. on wards or in a department
- Community settings, e.g. GP practices
- Drop-in centres, e.g. NHS walk-in centres

It is important for the nurse to begin to understand and build upon current knowledge regarding the types of intervention that can take place. In Table 4.5, Leach (2004) lists a range of some types of counselling interventions that may be available:

Table 4.5 Some types of counselling interventions

- Crisis intervention counselling
- Contact-based time limited counselling
- Ongoing counselling
- Advocacy and case work
- Assessment and referral

Source: Leach, 2004.

The crisis intervention approach

Crisis intervention is the only approach that will be briefly outlined in this chapter. There are various texts available that will help the nurse to develop a deeper understanding of the various approaches used when counselling.

Patients may often ask for help when they experience a crisis. During periods of crisis Parad and Parad (1990) suggest that brief interventions during crises can have a maximum effect, as opposed to other interventional approaches. A crisis can be caused by isolated events; often it is an accumulation of normal life events that are disruptive, produce stress, and may even bring on illness. Diagnosis of a sexually transmitted infection is an example of a situation that can precipitate a crisis for the individual with the diagnosis, the partner(s) and the family. The diagnosis of HIV can exacerbate a current life crisis such as a recent bereavement (Peate, 2004). A crisis, according to Hough (2003), can reactivate long-forgotten traumas or emotional problems from the past.

When faced with a crisis people will find themselves at a crossroads; they face problems and issues that they cannot deal with or rise above by using their usual coping mechanisms. Performing daily activities of living may be interrupted and become impossible to carry out as a result of the anxiety provoked by the crisis they face. The person may not be able to function effectively and they can often feel powerless to change their situation (Taylor et al., 2005).

Roberts (1995) defines crisis as a:

> temporary state of upset and disequilibrium characterized chiefly by an individual's inability to cope with a particular situation using existing methods of problem solving.

At the time a crisis can seem overwhelming to the patient; what one person perceives as crisis may not be seen as such by another – the experience of a crisis is subjective. Often it may be the crisis that brings the person into counselling for the first time. Those patients who may be in an immediate crisis situation may not wish to examine any other issue that underpins the crisis, e.g. relationships with other people; they may prefer to deal with the critical phase of the crisis, the 'here and now', and the energies of the counsellor should be directed at dealing with these immediate issues (Leach, 2004).

When helping the patient in crisis Hough (2003) suggests that the patient who comes forward for help is seeking the reassurance that somebody cares enough to intervene. What will help the patient is the identification of the patient's feelings and plans in order to conduct an assessment of risk. Having identified the risk, practical steps can be taken to lessen or reduce impact.

The following issues are considered important when working with people who are experiencing a crisis (Aguilera and Messick, 1982).

- The crisis intervention approach is the treatment of choice for some individuals.
- Accurate and rapid assessment of the presenting problem(s) and underlying factors is more important than a lengthy diagnostic evaluation.
- The treatment is sharply time limited and energies should be directed towards the resolution of the presenting problem working in the 'here and now' way.
- Time should not be wasted dealing with irrelevant material.
- There are occasions when a directive and active approach is needed to help the patient.
- Flexibility is key; there may be a need to act as resource provider, a co-ordinator and information giver.
- The goal of the intervention is to try to help the patient regain at least their pre-crisis level of functioning.

Undergoing an HIV test can instil fear and anxiety in some patients; some patients may view the situation as crisis. Below are some of the factors that the nurse needs to address and appreciate when providing pre- and post-HIV test counselling.

HIV testing

Those individuals who are to undergo, or are considering undergoing, testing for HIV will need special support and counselling. While this section of the chapter refers explicitly to issues surrounding HIV testing, the nurse may wish to consider applying the principles discussed here to other infections, for example hepatitis C testing.

Undergoing an HIV test should be done with the minimum of inconvenience to the patient. HIV testing is available from a variety of health care settings such as:

- GUM clinics;
- other hospital departments such as out-patients;
- open access same day testing clinics;
- private clinics;
- drug dependency clinics.

The support needed should occur prior to the test being undertaken and after the test has been taken – pre- and post-test counselling. This support is needed to help the individual understand and respond to the results.

The emotional and physical health of the patient can be affected by the results of the test. Often, it is not only the patient but also his/her family and friends who may be affected by the results. The nurse is able to empower the patient to make the right choice concerning the test.

The skills required to communicate with patients concerning sexual health issues have been addressed previously in this chapter and other chapters. The nurse must ensure that he/she possesses the appropriate skills necessary to discuss sensitive and intimate issues. Knowledge and understanding of contemporary developments in the domain of HIV/AIDS are also required as, regardless of the outcome of the test, the patient will need to have some understanding of the way the disease progresses, the range of treatments available and advice concerning safer sex.

Pre-test discussions

The Department of Health (DoH, 1996) states that there are three key reasons why a pre-test discussion is needed. In the first instance, the pre-test discussion can provide the patient with a chance to understand the reasons why the test is needed and why this applies to the patient. Secondly, it may help to ensure that the patient appreciates what information the test results will provide him/her with and the consequences of testing positive or negative, as well as the advantages and disadvantages of having the test. The third reason, as discussed by Ross and Channon-Little (2000), is that it provides the nurse and the patient with an opportunity to discuss preventative measures and how to instigate a reduction in risk-taking behaviours.

Pre-test counselling can be complex and several issues need to be addressed during the consultation. The Department of Health (DoH, 1996) suggest that the consultation should be made up of five key components (see Table 4.6).

Table 4.6 The five main components of pre-test counselling

- Ensuring that the individual understands the nature of HIV infection and that information about HIV transmission and risk is reduced
- Discussing activities that raise the risk of HIV infection, including the date of the last risk and the perception of the need for a test
- Discussing the benefits and difficulties for the individual and his/her family and associates of having a test and knowing the result, whether positive or negative
- Giving details of the test and how the result will be provided
- Obtaining an informed decision about whether or not to proceed with the test

Providing time for the patient is a vital aspect of pre- and post-HIV test counselling. There may be important issues that the patient may wish to raise. Ross and Channon-Little (2000) suggest that the nurse may need to allocate more time to the patient if it is his/her first attendance for having an HIV test. The nurse should be guided by the patient during the counselling session, as emphasis placed on different aspects of the discussion should be established by the needs of the individual patient (DoH, 1996).

Written information should also be provided to the patient in the pre-test discussion stage; such information is supplementary to the discussion. The nurse should be aware that there may be difficulties that arise during the consultation such as language difficulties, problems with comprehension or extreme anxiety, distress or embarrassment; if this does occur then it may be advisable to reschedule the appointment for another time (Peate, 2004).

It should be remembered that the Human Rights Act 1998, article 8 protects an individual's rights to respect for private and family life. Exceptional circumstances can occur where this right can be breached. The General Medical Council (1995) and Dimond (2005) state that breach may occur if the patient or another individual is at real risk of serious harm.

Structuring the test in a meaningful manner is important as the nurse needs to provide the patient with the information s/he requires. Pertinent questions should be asked, such as why s/he has attended and requested the test. In some instances the patient may refuse to state why they have requested a test; where this is the case this should be respected. The nurse should consider what is important and s/he must act in the patient's best interests (NMC, 2004a).

The reason why the patient has asked for an HIV test will determine if the following topics are appropriate for discussion:

- modes of transmission;
- the difference between infection with HIV and AIDS;
- ways in which transmission of the virus can be reduced.

The nurse needs to determine what is appropriate for discussion, and s/he does this by having insight and knowledge of the patient's circumstances and their reason for attending for the test. If, for example, a patient had been raped it would not be prudent – indeed it would be insensitive – to discuss modes of transmission; however, if the patient was an injecting drug user, discussion of modes of transmission may be acceptable and appropriate.

During the pre-test discussion the nurse should avoid making any statistical inferences; for example, a patient may be a male homosexual who by virtue of the statistical data is in a 'risk group', but he may be at no risk because of his sexual practices (Alder, 2001). It is the particular practices or behaviours that the nurse should ask the patient about that may have put him/her at risk. A discussion of risk groups is immaterial and even counterproductive to a discussion of risk behaviour with an individual.

Table 4.7 outlines some of the issues that the nurse needs to consider when conducting a pre-test HIV consultation.

Table 4.7 Issues that the nurse may wish to consider during the pre-test HIV consultation

- The patient's health
- The last date of involvement in risk-taking activity, such as unsafe sexual practice (for example anal/vaginal penetration, cunnilingus, fellatio, oro-anal activity)
- History of drug use and injecting exposure
- History of blood product use (e.g. factor VIII)
- History of blood transfusion prior to 1985 (before heat treating techniques)
- History of tattooing
- Occupation exposure (for example needlestick injury)
- History of overseas travel (e.g. travel to Sub-Saharan Africa) with exposure to risk activity

Source: Chippendale and French, 2001a.

A discussion concerning the advantages and disadvantages of taking an HIV test and the potential implications of a positive or negative result should take place. The nurse must establish what the patient thinks may be the main advantages and disadvantages of taking the test. The DoH (1996) outlines the advantages and disadvantages of taking an HIV test (see Table 4.8).

Table 4.8 Some of the possible advantages and disadvantages associated with taking an HIV test

Advantages	Disadvantages
Allows the individual to think about and formulate methods to protect any sexual partners. Provides safer sex information to avoid unsafe sexual activities	Knowledge of the result has the potential for an adverse impact on personal or professional relationships
Opportunity to provide information on sharing needles and syringes	
Allows interventions to reduce vertical transmission, for example referral to appropriate midwife/obstetrician. Women should be encouraged to discuss their special needs, e.g. breastfeeding	Psychological complications might arise from a positive result
Allows for appropriate medical interventions, e.g. referral to specialist HIV practitioner	Knowledge of the result might lead to restrictions on travel for those who test positive. Some countries require a declaration of freedom from HIV infection
Provides for effective prophylactic care, e.g. referral to specialist HIV practitioner	
Reduces any needless anxiety in the 'worried well'. Opportunity to provide support, advice and appropriate referrals	

An additional potential drawback of having an HIV test may be related to obtaining insurance. It may be more difficult to obtain insurance if the person has had an HIV test. The Association of British Insurers and the British Medical Association (2002) provide guidance on medical information and insurance.

At this stage it may be appropriate for the nurse to begin to investigate and ascertain how the patient may cope with a positive result. The nurse also needs to encourage the patient to start thinking about who s/he may want to tell if the result is positive; by doing this the nurse begins to help the patient to plan for the future.

Testing positive for HIV can generate a great deal of emotional and social distress; it can evoke a crisis in the patient and the result may put the patient or others at risk of harm. If a patient indicates that s/he may harm him/herself or another person as a result of the HIV test, then prior to the test being taken the nurse should work with the patient to achieve a realistic plan for coping (Ross and Channon-Little, 2000). The test may need to be postponed if this is the case, and the patient may have to be referred to an appropriate mental health professional. The following list gives details of other health care professionals to whom the patient may be referred in order to provide him/her with support:

• social worker
• psychiatrist
• clinical psychologist
• counsellor.

Attempting to determine what the patient's response to the outcome of the test may be can alert the nurse to the need for support before or after the test has been conducted. The nurse needs to be aware of his/her limitations, for example, if the patient has a known psychiatric illness such as previous suicide attempts, suicidal idealization or psychosis the pre-test counselling session may be better undertaken by a health care practitioner with mental health expertise. After the test has been concluded it is important that there is adequate psychiatric follow-up available (Ross and Channon-Little, 2000).

If the nurse is aware of a recent (within the last twelve months) life crisis that might have occurred, for example, the death of a loved one, Ross and Channon-Little (2000) suggest that the patient may find that a positive HIV test outcome can exacerbate any ongoing problems that the patient may be experiencing in relation to the life crisis. The nurse therefore needs to gather together as much information about the patient as possible to plan the strategies needed to cope with a positive HIV test outcome.

An explanation of the test is needed; the nurse will be expected to adhere to local policy and procedure when undertaking diagnostic tests.

The explanation should include details about when and how the results will be given to the patient. Prior to undertaking the test the nurse should ensure that the patient gives his/her consent; this means that the nurse must provide the patient with enough information to make an informed decision. The complex issue of informed consent is discussed elsewhere – for example, Department of Health (2001a). The patient's consent to undertake the test should be documented in his/her notes.

The information contained in Table 4.9 regarding HIV, its transmission, progression and potential treatment should also be provided to the patient verbally and supplemented in a written form, as any information given to the patient may not be retained or recalled as the patient may be in a state of shock.

Table 4.9 Supplementary health education information to be offered to the patient concerning HIV and its transmission

---

- A positive test indicates that the patient is infected and as such is infectious and will probably remain infected for the rest of his/her life
- An HIV positive patient is infectious to others where there is transfer of:
  - Blood
  - Semen
  - Vaginal fluid
- The individual should practice safer sex activities, for example the use of condoms, and reduce the risk of transferring infected body fluids

---

Source: Ross and Channon-Little, 2000.

Post-test discussions

The nurse must be aware that any information given to the patient in a post-test discussion context may not be retained or remembered (as is the case in the pre-test context) as the patient may be highly anxious or in a state of shock on receiving a positive result, or conversely in a state of elation if s/he receives a negative test result. These psychological states may overwhelm any information or advice given.

If at all possible, the same health care professional who conducted the pre-test discussion should preferably also conduct the post-test discussions with the patient DoH (2002a).

Ideally, during the pre-test discussions phase the nurse should have provided the patient with a date and time for the post-test consultation concerning the time when s/he will receive the test results. Regardless of the outcome of the test, i.e. a positive or negative result, all patients should receive post-test counselling; no test results should be given out over the telephone.

A negative result

A negative test result means that HIV antibodies have not been detected. Usually, this means that the patient is not infected or that s/he remains in the 'window period', for example, that s/he has not been involved in possible exposure to the virus for the last six months. If the patient is in the 'window period' the DoH (1996) recommend that a repeat test be performed in three to six months; the patient will also need pre- and post-test counselling at the subsequent tests.

The primary aim of the post-test counselling discussion, when the patient has tested negative, is to reinforce and clarify health education concerning safer sex, condom use and injecting equipment. An opportunity will exist for the nurse to reiterate how the virus is transmitted and offer the patient a chance to seek clarification of issues discussed at the pre-test session, or any other issues that may have arisen since that session.

A positive result

Being diagnosed with HIV is one of the most significant life events that an individual may face (National Aids Manual (NAM), 2004). Time must be set aside to allow the patient to react to the news that the test has proved positive. The time needed will depend upon the patient's reaction to the result. It is difficult to predict the emotions or feelings the patient may experience after the diagnosis has been made. NAM (2004) reports that some common reactions and feelings are:

* numbness
* frightened
* upset
* tearful
* desperate
* angry.

Some people have also felt relieved to have finally found out.

Chippendale and French (2001b) suggest that giving the HIV result is similar to giving the result of any test relating to any chronic illness and the nurse is adept at providing test results. For the patient there may be both physical and psychological consequences; s/he may need more help and support than the nurse is able to provide. Discussion concerning the implications for the future should be addressed, including the immediate future and beyond, and the patient should be encouraged to talk about these important issues. The nurse needs to be knowledgeable about the range of agencies that s/he may have to refer the patient to; this knowledge must be available prior to the post-test consultation.

It is not easy breaking the news to the patient that the test is positive, but the nurse must not prevaricate. If it is perceived by the patient that the nurse has difficulties in dealing with the result, then this will not instil confidence in the patient.

There must be a balance between providing the patient with hope when the result is known and providing false reassurances. There are and have been, and will be, significant advances and developments in drug therapies and the long-term management of HIV-infected people. People with HIV are now living longer (Chippendale and French, 2001a). Finding out that the test result is positive can put the patient in a position that will encourage him/her to start taking steps to begin looking after their health (NAM, 2004). The sooner HIV infection is diagnosed the sooner the patient can (if they decide to) receive the appropriate care. The nurse should avoid telling the patient that everything will be fine and not to worry – HIV remains a disease without a cure.

Effective, compassionate and sensitive interpersonal skills are essential when communicating the result to the patient. The nurse needs to be aware of what the patient is trying to communicate – not only their verbal responses but also non-verbal responses; time must be given over to the patient to talk through issues that may arise. Coming to terms with the diagnosis may take longer for some individuals than others. The patient may, when coming to terms with the result, begin to ask fundamental questions such as:

- What is the difference between HIV and AIDS?
- How long will it be before I die?
- How long does it take before I become ill?
- Do I have to pay for my treatments (i.e. prescriptions)?

The patient for the first time may come across various medical terms that are new to them and they may not understand them; the nurse can provide that understanding by explaining clearly, supplementing this with written information. For many patients this is the first time they have ever had any prolonged contact with the health service and health service practitioners; all of this will be new to them and may be a perplexing experience for them.

At this stage it may not be advisable to provide information about HIV and HIV disease as the patient may be too distressed to understand and assimilate. The nurse needs to use his/her professional judgement here. Offer the patient contact numbers. Some patients may wish to use these, others may not. Follow-up appointments are needed and this will depend on local policy and practice. The patient may prefer to see his/her GP or a specialist to plan care and treatment.

Concluding the session or terminating the encounter also needs to be done effectively and with sensitivity, e.g.:

• reassurance that a practitioner will continue to assist the patient;
• confirmation that a follow-up appointment has been made;
• an expression of personal support.

Table 4.10 summarizes some of the key issues that the nurse might address during a post-test discussion.

Table 4.10 Key issues to be addressed during the post-test discussion

• Address the patient's immediate reactions
• Refer for specialist management (consider both physical and psychological support)
• Provide details of support services
• Offer follow-up appointments

Any discussion concerning HIV and the possibility of the patient requesting an HIV test must be handled competently and confidently. The nurse's interpersonal skills can have an impact on how the patient responds to, and comes to terms with, the result of the test.

This aspect of the chapter has provided the reader with advice concerning pre- and post-test counselling. The nurse will also need to seek support to help him/her deal with the emotions that may be associated with the provision of HIV test results.

Supervision

Support and supervision are an important aspect of coping with emotional stress and tensions. Supervision refers to the practice of giving support and guidance to counsellors who work with patients (Hough, 2003). Regular planned contact with others, or another person who is working in the field of sexual health and sexual health counselling, is advocated and the aim of this interaction is to share and learn from difficult or painful situations. Clinical supervision is an integral aspect of developing and enhancing counselling skills; some aspects and reasons for supervision can be summarized as:

• the sharing of ideas with others;
• providing an objective view of the counsellor's work;
• reducing 'burnout';
• promoting the use of reflection in order to appraise the skills and approaches used with individual patients;

- providing time for reflection;
- passing on useful information about contacts and helpful resources;
- giving attention to colleagues who appear overloaded or distressed;
- supporting each other in order to be able to provide more support to the patient (Lindon and Lindon, 2000; Hough, 2003).

It is necessary for the nurse to regularly reflect on his/her practice; the use of supervision can provide the vehicle for this to occur. Supervision is not therapy for the nurse but has the potential to provide therapeutic benefits. The primary aim of the supervisory encounter is to improve the nurse's relationship with the patient. Clinical supervision complements other kinds of supervision and other forms of support available to the nurse in the workplace. The supervisor should not be the nurse's line manager; s/he should be an external expert practitioner.

The worried well patient

There are some patients the nurse may see who present with multiple pathology, and the patient may interpret multiple physical complaints as signs of HIV infection, sexually transmitted infection or some other illness (Jarrett, 2004). Often they are not reassured that the signs and symptoms they are presenting with are not associated with an STI or HIV, and their feelings and fears of infection can reach obsessive proportions.

Bor et al. (1993) and Chippendale and French (2001a) provide a list of characteristics that can be associated with the 'worried well' patient:

- repeated negative tests and investigations;
- low-risk sexual history, including covert and guilt-inducing sexual activity;
- socially isolated;
- experienced/experiencing relationship problems;
- multiple misinterpreted physical (somatic) features;
- a psychiatric history;
- repeated consultations with GPs/practice nurses;
- evidence of anxiety, depression and obsessive behaviour;
- misunderstanding of health education messages.

Referral should always be made to a doctor if the nurse deems this appropriate so that any current or outstanding medical issues are dealt with. Exclusion of the physical illness is vital (Bor et al., 1998).

Spending time with the patient listening to his/her concerns and anxieties may resolve a patient's worry. However, not all patients will be reassured, even when on repeated occasions tests have come back negative;

in this instance the nurse may need to refer the patient to another appropriate health care professional. Bor et al. (1998) state that at all costs the patient should not be labelled:

- hypochondriacal
- compulsive
- obsessive
- hysterical.

To care for the 'worried well' patient the nurse needs to have the necessary skills and experiences to provide the most appropriate care. Jarrett (2004) recommends that if the nurse does not posses these skills she/he must refer the patient to a clinical psychologist or psychiatrist.

Conclusion

This chapter has provided the reader with a brief overview of the counselling skills needed by the nurse in order to support a patient with an STI. The complex issues associated with information giving, offering advice and support provision have been discussed.

Key terms have been defined and discussed in an endeavour to define what is meant by counselling and to differentiate between counselling, using counselling skills and using communication skills. Nurses use a variety of skills to give advice to patients in a professional manner on a variety of social problems; a number of these skills have been described and discussed. Some nurses may be counsellors and can counsel patients; the majority of nurses are not counsellors. However, nurses can develop and use therapeutic communication and therapeutic nursing interventions to help the patient identify their own problems and seek resources to deal with these problems, and the nurse aims to empower the patient.

There are at least 300–400 models of counselling and psychotherapy from which to choose. The type of intervention will depend very much on the nurse's skills, the patient, and the content of care. Evidence-based guidance has been produced by the Department of Health to help the practitioner determine the most appropriate intervention.

The crisis intervention approach has been briefly outlined as one approach that may be appropriate when caring for a patient with an STI. A discussion has been presented that outlines the care of a patient who may undergo HIV testing. Pre- and post-test counselling is an obligatory requirement and often it is the nurse who conducts this. Primary care settings, for example, are appropriate locations in which to offer HIV tests and as such pre- and post-test counselling will also be needed. Informed consent is an issue that must be given serious consideration prior to conducting the test. The nurse must provide the patient with information that alerts them to the implications of a positive or negative result.

Providing the patient with an HIV positive test result can be traumatic for both the nurse and the patient. The nurse needs support in order to develop coping mechanisms; clinical supervision may be one way in which this support can be provided. Clinical supervision is a regular planned event and exists in order to provide support and guidance to those who work with patients. The clinical supervisor should be a knowledgeable experienced practitioner.

The nurse may encounter patients referred to as the 'worried well'; these patients will also require skilled nursing care. The patient presents with multiple physical complaints often convinced that they are STI related; the feelings and fear of contagion can be so strong as to be obsessive. The nurse may need to refer this patient to the most appropriate health care professional.

The counselling process is intended to facilitate and enable the patient to make his/her own decisions or be able to help him/her to adapt to the challenge which he/she faces. Whether counselling or using counselling skills, the nurse will respect the patient's values, choices and lifestyle.

CHAPTER FIVE

Partner notification

Introduction

The term 'partner notification' has generally replaced the term 'contact tracing'. As a rule partner notification is most appropriate as it reflects the ideal, in so far as the patient informs their partner(s) themselves. However, Faldon (2004a) proposes that the terms are frequently used interchangeably and are often used to convey identical meaning. Potterat et al. (1998) suggest that 'partner notification' can be described as the shell of the context but 'contact tracing' the soul.

Gibson and Mindel (2001) report that failure to treat partners of those with an STI is often a common cause of 'treatment failure'. Macke and Maher (1999) and Matthews and Fletcher (2001) indicate from an international perspective that partner notifications are an effective means of detecting new infections and that more partners are notified and medically evaluated when compared to self-referral. Partner notification when concerned with HIV infection was more effective than for STIs (Mathews et al., 2003).

Partner notification is often carried out by health advisors who work predominantly in the GUM clinic. Despite this there may be occasions where the nurse or other health care practitioners may have to assume this role, or it could be that the nurse is the most appropriate person to carry out partner notification in certain situations. The issue of partner notification concerns all health care professionals, particularly those within the primary care arena:

- specialist community public health nurses;
- practice nurses;
- community nurses;
- health visitors;
- school nurses;
- midwives;

- infection control nurses;
- sexual health nurses;
- general practitioners.

Without doubt the nurse has an overriding responsibility to the patient and is accountable to the patient first and foremost (NMC, 2004a). However, when becoming involved with the management and care of people with STIs some responsibility is also owed to the health and well-being of sexual partners and other contacts of the patient. The responsibility has to be balanced against the patient's right to care and confidentiality and community sensitivities that are associated with the importance of public health. Legal and ethical concerns are addressed in Chapter 6.

The development of policy concerning the complex and sensitive issue of partner notification requires an integrated approach. If policy is to be responsive and sensitive to need – reducing the spread of infection – there must be representation from various stakeholders:

- a range of health care professionals;
- affected communities;
- government.

Some of the key objectives associated with partner notification are shown in Table 5.1.

Table 5.1 Some objectives related to partner notification

- To interrupt the transmission of infection
- To identify people with an infection who may benefit from treatment
- To identify people with an infection and offer treatment in order to minimize complications of infection
- To offer individual counselling to promote sustained behaviour change among the infected patient or people at risk of infection

Partner notification that is undertaken by inexperienced people in an insensitive manner has the potential to alienate individuals and whole communities. If the process of partner notification is not done with sensitivity by an experienced practitioner then the objectives described above will not be met. In order to achieve the above objectives the practitioner must be knowledgeable; being aware of the ethical and legal implications, s/he should act in a professional manner and assess each case individually, taking into account the biopsychosocial aspects of the patient's circumstances. It may be difficult and complex to obtain consent to contact others when, for example, the infection has been acquired from a relationship not sanctioned by the group or religion (Wakley et al., 2003).

The principles underpinning partner notification should take into account the serious medical, social, public health, ethical and legal issues involved in a comprehensive control programme. In Table 5.2 the underlying principles have been identified.

Table 5.2 The general principles underpinning partner notification

- The patient's human rights should be respected and protected
- Partner notification is only one aspect of prevention and care
- Partner notification should be carried out on a voluntary basis and without coercion
- The process should be confidential
- Partner notification should only be undertaken when there are adequate and appropriate services available to the index case and his/her contact(s)

This chapter will discuss the important issue of partner notification. The rationale underpinning this activity and how it plays an important role in reducing the incidence of STIs is also included. Practical advice is offered on how partner notification can be performed.

Definitions

Partner notification and contact tracing

Earlier it has been identified that the definition of terms is important. According to Faldon (2004a) it is more than a semantic argument and is worthy of further discussion. Partner notification used as a tool in the fight against infection can help to control infection and in so doing alerts the unsuspecting. It is suggested that the term 'partner' can mean and imply a degree of commitment to a relationship; 'contact' does not. However, it must be remembered that not all patients have partners; furthermore the term 'partner' excludes those who share needles, and therefore, in some respects the term is rather narrow. Patterns of sexual mixing and the sexual partner network are important determinants of the spread of all STIs. Ghani et al. (1997) believe that the term contact tracing has been rekindled as this may have epidemiological implications.

Partner notification and contact tracing are the process of identifying relevant contacts of a person with a sexually transmitted infection, ensuring that they are aware of their exposure. Contact is made with the individual with whom the index person has had sex during the infectious period. Partner notification and contact tracing can also be used in the process of contacting persons with other infections, for example tuberculosis.

Patient, partner, passive or self-referral

The index patient (this is the patient who was the original person identified with the infection, who may or may not have infected other persons but represents a starting point for the process of tracing) informs the sexual partner(s). The person is encouraged to notify the partner(s) of the possible infection without any involvement of the health care services or personnel. Faldon (2004a) recommends that the patient may:

- provide the partner with information;
- accompany the partner to the clinic;
- hand over a contact slip (the slip and the contents of the slip may be provided by the health care worker).

Initially there is no third party involvement.

Provider or active referral

In this instance it is the health care worker who notifies the patient's partner(s). The index person provides information concerning the partner(s) to the health care worker who then goes about confidentially tracing and notifying the partner(s) directly. This approach requires third party involvement.

Conditional, contract or negotiated referral

If the contact has not attended the GUM clinic, for example, the initial patient referral is followed up by a provider referral after a certain period of time; this is a hybrid approach (Faldon, 2004a). The condition is the agreed period of time.

Partner management

This term may be seen as a more 'holistic' expression and according to Faldon (2004a) is an amalgam of the terms 'partner notification' and 'contact tracing'.

Partner notification – the process

Just as the nurse needs to use counselling skills to provide the patient with advice and support, the use of effective counselling skills is equally important when undertaking a partner notification exercise. Partner notification is a complex and challenging activity; the health care professional who is considering undertaking this activity must be experienced, confident and competent. If the nurse feels unable to undertake partner notification then the patient must be referred to a specialist practitioner who possesses the necessary skills.

The positive outcome of partner notification relies upon the goodwill and cooperation of the patient (the index case). No person (in the case of STIs) can be forced to attend for treatment or to make known the names and other details of contacts. For partner notification to work the health care practitioner undertaking the activity must be non-judgemental and supportive. As well as possessing counselling skills the following attributes are required:

- tact;
- empathy;
- awareness and understanding.

The health care practitioner must use effective interviewing skills (including the way the interview is structured and techniques employed) to reduce resistance and to promote participation. Bell (2004b) states that all patients with an STI that may result in significant morbidity in an untreated partner may be referred. The range of infections can include:

- gonorrhoea
- chlamydia
- syphilis
- HIV
- hepatitis B
- hepatitis C
- non-specific urethritis.

If partner notification is to work effectively and ultimately result in a reduction in STIs then all members of the health care team (e.g. GP practice) must be supportive of this activity. The aim should be to make the patient's experience a positive experience. The encounter may well impact on the patient and could result in him/her agreeing to an interview. An efficient internal referral system must be in place. In order to secure the interview regarding partner notification the following points have been suggested by Bell (2004b):

- All staff should understand the rationale, process and importance of partner notification.
- All staff should understand their specific role in the process of partner notification.

- Waiting times for the referral are kept to a minimum.
- Patients are managed appropriately.
- Patients are treated with warmth and respect.

The timing of the interview to discuss partner notification should be timed to occur after diagnosis and treatment have commenced. When the interview occurs at this stage it allows the health care professional to clarify issues surrounding all aspects of care. Some patients will not be prepared to wait until after the diagnosis and treatment have been given; if this is the case it may be beneficial to work with the patient when the treatment is being dispensed. The most appropriate time to embark on the contact tracing process will need to be judged on a case by case basis. However, there are certain factors that will influence this decision and some of these have been highlighted in Table 5.3.

Table 5.3 Some factors to take into account regarding initiation of the contact tracing process

- The patient's psychological and physical state – it may be better to leave the contact tracing interview until another time if there is acute physical and/or mental distress

- The patient's priority – for some patients the notifying of contacts may be highest on their agenda and it may be beneficial to deal with this immediately

- The nature of the condition. In highly infectious conditions such as chlamydia and gonorrhoea that can be treated relatively easily, the process of contact tracing is often dealt with when the index patient has been diagnosed and treatment has commenced. In infections that are chronic and viral in nature the contact tracing process can be deferred. This allows the patient, during this acute stage, time to come to terms with the diagnosis and treatment options

- Public health factors – when it is considered that the patient is putting others at immediate risk of infection, contact tracing is urgent

Source: adapted from Australasian Society for HIV Medicine, 2002.

To proceed with the interview effectively, good preparation is needed to ensure that the outcome is a positive one. Bell (2004b) recommends that the following background points should be known prior to meeting and beginning the process with the patient (see Table 5.4). Doing this allows the discussion to be modified and adapted to the patient's individual needs.

Chapter 2 (regarding the taking of a sexual health history) has already emphasized the importance of ensuring that the environment must be conducive to allowing the patient to reveal as much or as little as they wish, the

Table 5.4 Background information needed before beginning the contact tracing process with the patient

- The reason for attendance, e.g. was this a routine check-up? does the patient have any symptoms? who referred the patient – was it his/her partner or another agency, e.g. the patient's GP practice nurse?
- What are the symptoms, the duration and type?
- Sexual health history
- The outcome of investigations and any treatment prescribed
- Concerns or issues the patient may have
- Details of known contacts i.e.
  - Name
  - Diagnosis
  - Date attended/treated
  - Sexual health history

Source: adapted from Bell, 2004b.

patient must be made to feel safe and supported. The health care professional has to be open with the patient and in so doing set aside any fears of being judged or interrogated; the purpose of the interview should be made clear, offering the patient support, respect and if so required, advice. Avoid being uninterested, shocked or irritated as these negative signals will hamper a response. Initially the patient's needs must be addressed. By giving the patient priority it conveys to the patient that he/she is being respected and treated as an individual.

Open-ended questions are needed in order to facilitate disclosure, for example:

- 'How do you think you might have picked up the infection?'
- 'Who do you think you might need to tell about your condition?'
- 'Who else do you think may be involved?'
- 'How do you think your partner(s) might react?'
- 'How long do you think you have had the infection?'

Avoid questions such as:

- 'Who might you have given this to?'
- 'Is there anybody else you could have infected?'

Assessing the patient's understanding can be done more effectively by using open-ended questions. A skilled assessment is vital at this stage as it can prevent patronizing the patient and can also disclose many other things about the patient, for example:

- his/her cognitive level;

- preferred language;
- level of fear/anxiety.

As there is no statutory requirement in the UK for a patient to disclose and identify partner(s) (Cowan et al., 1996), the patient must be motivated to participate and engage fully in the interview. It may be useful to motivate the patient by explaining to him/her about the risks associated with leaving an infection untreated, emphasizing that the contact may be asymptomatic and therefore unaware of the infection. Reassure the patient that all aspects of the interview are confidential and the contact will not be told about their infection or their partners.

A rapport must be developed whereby the patient feels listened to and, as such, a part of the decision-making process, in control and empowered. Offer the patient choice and reassurance that he/she will not be forced into doing anything he/she does not wish to do or anything against their will. The encounter must be

- non-threatening;
- free from coercion;
- free from bullying;
- free from feelings of being blackmailed;
- non-discriminatory;
- non-prejudicial.

Asking the patient where s/he thinks s/he may have picked up the infection may prompt them to offer names or volunteer more important details. Bell (2004b) suggests that the patient should be invited to 'set the scene'. General terms should be used, as most patients at this initial stage are willing to talk in general terms and to use first names of contacts; asking non-threatening question such as 'where did you meet?' may provide information about the patient's social and sexual scene/setting, i.e. type of sexual activity engaged in, gender and relationship. Having begun to establish this important aspect of the encounter, it may help to understand the patient's values, attitudes, language and behaviours associated with transmission (Potterat et al., 1985).

Using the social context to trace a contact can also be fruitful. By learning more about where people meet can uncover, according to Potterat et al. (1985), key locations that may be functional to transmission, for example particular pubs/clubs, saunas, drug houses (e.g. crack dens, shooting galleries). Being aware of these key locations can give opportunities to offer health promotion and other additional control efforts (Woodhouse et al., 1987; Bell and Brady, 2000). Furthermore, Hopkins et al. (2001) suggest that this 'social context awareness' can also provide the opportunity for on-site screening to take place.

People with multiple sexual partners may forget a considerable proportion of their partners, and drug injectors can also forget a large number of the persons with whom they inject drugs (Brewer et al., 1999). Such incomplete reports can hinder contact tracing; Brewer and Garrett (2001) have used and evaluated memory prompts that are practical adjuncts that may help the patient who has multiple partners to recall those partners s/he may have forgotten. Table 5.5 describes the memory prompts advocated by Brewer and Garrett (2001).

Table 5.5 Memory prompts that can be used in encouraging patients to recall forgotten individuals

Role cues
- These cues focus on the types of relationships mentioned by the patient. These may include:
  - Regular partner(s)
  - Casual partner(s)
  - Ex partners(s)
  - One-night stand(s)
  - Client(s)
  - Dealer(s)
  - Sex worker(s)

The interviewer should ask the patient to consider if there is anybody else with whom she/he has a relationship

Location cues
- These require the patient to recall where they met each named contact and then to consider who else they have met at each of the locations mentioned

Personal timeline cues
- Personal timeline cues involve the indication of key events during the lookback period, for example:
  - Holidays
  - Business trips (abroad or in the UK)
  - Time spent in prison (including for example detention centres)
  - The end of a relationship

Having considered these key events the patient is then asked to think about sexual contact associated with each event

Network cues
- Focus is made on the partners already identified. The patient is then asked to consider whether they have had sex with anyone else known to each named contact

Alphabetic cues
- Ask the patient to recall as well as they can all recent partners whose name begins with A, B, C, ... each letter of the alphabet

Source: adapted from Brewer and Garrett, 2001.

The use of such cues has been subjected to evaluation using randomized control (Brewer and Garrrett, 2001). These supplementary techniques have been shown to encourage remembering and noticeably counteract forgetting and may promote more effective partner notification and a more complete description of risk networks.

Notifying the contact

Patient referral has already been discussed. The patient notifies the partner themselves or the patient allows the health care professional to do this without the patient's name being revealed (provider referral). Conditional referral can also be used where a provider referral is initiated if the patient has not attended by an agreed time.

Contacts may be advised by either *patient referral* or *provider referral*.

Patient referral

Preparing for the notification is important and it may be advisable to discuss with the patient how s/he intends to inform the contact – where and when. The patient will be encouraged to think about the most appropriate place, time and the choice of words to be used. The patient must be well informed and confident in approaching the contact; the health care worker can rehearse, e.g. role play, this with the patient if s/he lacks confidence.

The most appropriate choice of informing will depend on specific circumstances. The following approaches can be used:

* face to face;
* by telephone;
* by post;
* in a pre-destined meeting place, e.g. pub/club.

The health care provider may also provide a contact slip to pass to the contact and this details information regarding the infection and treatment (Appendix 5.1 details the content of a contact slip).

Provider referral

The way the contact is approached will depend on the quality and the amount of information the patient has provided. Regardless of what approach is used the explicit approval of the patient must be given. Provider referral may offer the patient a higher level of confidentiality. The following approaches may be considered:

- telephone;
- post;
- personal visit.

The health care worker should be guided by the patient with regard to the most appropriate approach to use. Provider referral is resource intensive and can be time-consuming. Table 5.6 highlights the advantages and disadvantages associated with provider referral.

Table 5.6 Some of the advantages and disadvantages associated with provider referral

	Advantages	Disadvantages
Telephone	Saves time and allows for an appointment to be organized Cost effective Confidential Some anxiety can be allayed	Provides verbal cues only Inappropriate disclosure of full details Can be intercepted by a third person Inappropriate for the contact who speaks no English or is hearing impaired
Letter	After the contact has received the letter allows them to phone when their confidentiality has been assured The letter may be redirected if the person is not at home or has moved	May create anxiety if the contact receives the letter and services are closed May be intercepted by a third person Of little value to those contacts who have literacy difficulties
Visit	The health care worker is able to give full details immediately, deal with the response and provide links with appropriate support networks Can offer on-the-spot testing (if appropriate)	Being visible can detract from providing confidentiality May be interpreted as 'policing' Expensive and time consuming

Source: adapted from Australasian Society for HIV Medicine, 2002.

There may be instances when the patient refuses to provide details concerning contacts. The health care worker in this instance would be advised to speak again with the patient to ascertain the reasons why they may be so reluctant. In some cases the patient may reconsider if s/he is offered support; a positive outcome may often hinge on the skills of the health care worker providing partner notification advice. It may be that time is all that is needed for the patient to reconsider and to develop trust between the patient and the health care worker.

If the patient is truly uncooperative, then a balance must be made between respecting the patient's rights, preserving confidentiality, and protecting public health. A balance must be made between providing a duty to warn, a duty of care and duty to maintain confidentiality.

Table 5.7 outlines some of the reasons why a patient may be reluctant to cooperate with the health care provider and offers some suggested strategies.

Table 5.7 Some reasons why a patient may not want to cooperate with the health care provider and some suggested strategies

Reason	Suggested strategies
Fear of loss of confidentiality	May prefer the use of provider referral thereby providing a higher level of confidentiality
Unassertive patient	Practise role play to build up confidence
Patient unaware of the seriousness of the consequences for his/her contacts	Educate the patient
Patient has little concern for consequences to contacts	Explain that contacts tend to find out anyway as another patient may name the same contact. Re-advise about the risks of re-infection There may be a case for notifying the contact without the patient's consent

Source: adapted from Australasian Society for HIV Medicine, 2002.

The use of the Internet for partner notification

The most common methods of partner notification have been discussed above. One further approach that has not received much comment is the use of the Internet to inform contacts.

Toomey and Rothenberg (2000) have estimated that one-third of people visiting the Internet aged 18 years or over do so to access sexually oriented websites, chat rooms and news groups that allow users to view sexual images or to take part in online sexual discussion. While cyberspace sex carries no risk of transmitting an STI it can act as a vehicle to meet sexual partners and the outcome of that liaison may carry with it the risk of transmission. The use of the Internet therefore can become a sexually risk-taking behaviour (Klausner et al., 2000).

McFarlene at al. (2000) note that the Internet allows anonymity by allowing participants to withhold identifying information such as:

- full name
- address
- place of employment.

As a result of this it may pose challenges for those health care workers who attempt to undertake partner notification. The Internet has already been used to notify sexual partners of persons with STIs: Pioquinto et al. (2004) describe two instances (reported from the USA) where the Internet was used successfully to contact partners who would otherwise have remained anonymous. Therefore it may be that policy development teams consider the Internet as another addition to their repertoire of methods used to notify partners.

In one reported case a patient had reported 16 sex partners all of whom he had met via the Internet during the infectious period; he subsequently tested positive for syphilis. He was asked to inform his contacts via email regarding the infection. He was able to supply the health care provider with the 16 email addresses and copies of emails he had sent them. Seven of the contacts replied and made arrangements to be tested for syphilis. This case demonstrates that the use of an email via the patient has the potential to improve partner response rates.

Further research is needed in order to determine the true effectiveness of the Internet as another method of partner notification. It is important that the health care worker remembers that the same confidentiality rules apply to messages sent via the telephone or in the post as those messages sent over the Internet. Table 5.8 provides some guidance for partner notification online.

Partner notification recommendations

Often the term 'lookback period' is used to determine how far back the health care worker needs to trace back the contacts of the index case. Wakley et al. (2003) suggest that usually the sexual contacts who are notified are:

- all sexual partners in the last four weeks of people with symptoms;
- all sexual partners within the last six months or the most recent sexual partner(s) of people with no symptoms.

Below (Table 5.9) are the partner notification recommendations suggested by Faldon (2004a) and Australasian Society of HIV Medicine (2002); these recommendations refer to the nine STIs discussed in Chapter 3.

Table 5.8 Guidance for partner notification online

- If the original patient notifies his/her partner first, the likelihood of the partner responding to the health care worker might be increased
- Messages sent from within the Internet Service Provider (ISP) or email provider are less likely to be discarded before being read. If the partner's email account is provided through company X, a company X account should be used to send the message
- Credible email accounts (e.g. those with a .gov domain) should be used. Specific, verifiable information about the sender should be provided within the email message
- Message headers that reference a serious health matter are more likely to be read than general messages. However, messages should not mention that a person has been exposed to an STI. Message headers should convey urgency but protect confidentiality (e.g. 'Urgent Health Matter')
- A message should be sent to each partner individually; no group messages should be sent. To protect confidentiality, notification procedures should apply the same principles used in sending a letter in the mail or leaving a telephone message
- When a person responds, name and alternative locating information should be obtained to facilitate contact in future

Source: adapted from Kent et al., 2003.

Table 5.9 Lookback and implications for partner notification

Infection	Recommendations	Comments
Gonorrhoea	Partner notification required According to sexual history, up to six months	• Sexual partners exposed by vaginal, anal or oral sex without using a condom are at highest risk. These contacts should be screened for gonorrhoea and chlamydial infections • Men with urethral symptoms, two weeks before the onset of symptoms • Men without symptoms and all women, twelve weeks prior to diagnosis at urethra, cervix, rectum and throat • If a patient's last sexual intercourse was more than eight weeks before onset of symptoms or diagnosis, the patient's most recent sex partner is to be treated
Syphilis	Partner notification required	• Patients should be encouraged to refer sexual partners and contacts

Table 5.9 continued

Infection	Recommendations	Comments
Syphilis	This will depend on the stage of the infection and how it was acquired Early syphilis: 12 weeks (primary) Up to 2 years (secondary) Late syphilis: Vertical transmission can be as long as 10 years post-infection Gummata – 2 years Cardiovascular – 10 years Neurological – 15 years	for evaluation and treatment. The patient should be offered provider referral • After the first year of infection transmission is uncommon • Any person exposed sexually to a person with syphilis regardless of the stage should be referred for clinical evaluation

Chlamydia	Partner notification required
	According to sexual history, up to six months
		• Patients should be encouraged to refer sexual partners and contacts for evaluation and treatment. The patient should be offered provider referral
		• Sexual partners exposed by vaginal, anal or oral sex without using a condom are at highest risk. These contacts should be screened for gonorrhoea and chlamydial infections
		• Partner(s) should be treated regardless of the symptoms or test result
		• The following criteria should be used for sexual contacts:
		  – 4 weeks prior to the onset of symptoms in men
		  – 6 months or until the last previous partner (whichever is the longer time period) for all women and asymptomatic men

Non-specific urethritis	Partner notification required	• Patients should be encouraged to refer sexual partners and contacts for evaluation and treatment. The patient should be offered provider referral • The following criteria should be used for sexual contacts:

Table 5.9 continued

Infection	Recommendations	Comments
Non-specific urethritis (contd)		– 4 weeks prior to the onset of symptoms in men – 6 months or until the last previous partner (whichever is the longer time period) for all women and asymptomatic men • Ideally, details regarding contacts should be obtained at the first visit with consent to contact the partner(s) if tests for chlamydia or gonorrhoea are positive
Trichomonas	Partner notification required Lookback to current partner	• Patients should be encouraged to refer sexual partners and contacts for evaluation and treatment. The patient should be offered provider referral
Genital herpes	Not offered routinely	• Limited therapeutic intervention • May be advisable to offer support or counselling to partner(s)
Genital warts	Not offered routinely	• No evidence to suggest that partner notification reduces transmission or prevents re-infection • May be advisable to offer current partners screening for other STIs
HIV	Partner notification required Lookback period will depend on risk assessment and previous testing results May need to look back as far as 1980 for late HIV infection or an infection of unknown duration	• Patients should be encouraged to refer sexual partners and contacts for evaluation and treatment. The patient should be offered provider referral
Hepatitides	Partner notification required	
	HAV	• Patient or provider referral offered to male homosexual contacts from

Table 5.9 continued

Infection	Recommendations	Comments
Hepatitides	HAV	two weeks before to one week after onset of jaundice • At-risk non-sexual contacts such as household contacts, referred to Public Health Authorities and/or the Health Protection Agency
	HBV	• Patient or provider referral offered to any sexual contact (penetrative vaginal or anal sex) or needle-sharing partners from 2 weeks before onset of jaundice until blood tests are surface antigen negative • Risk assessment required for asymptomatic cases • Screening required for children who have been born to infectious women if the child was not vaccinated at birth • At-risk non-sexual contacts such as household contacts, referred to Public Health Authorities and/or the Health Protection Agency
	HCV	• Patient or provider referral offered to any sexual contact (penetrative vaginal or anal sex) or needle-sharing partners during period of infectivity – 2 weeks before onset of jaundice • Risk assessment required for asymptomatic cases • Consider testing children born to infectious women • Non-sexual contacts such as household contacts, referred to Public Health Authorities and/or the Health Protection Agency

Source: Faldon, 2004a and Australasian Society for HIV Medicine, 2002.

Special needs populations

There are challenges concerning patient notification for all sections of society (including the index patient and his/her contact(s)) such as fear of retaliation or reprisal, anxiety concerning prosecution and a fear of disclosure. Effective partner notification clearly depends on the patient's accurate disclosure of the names and contact details of all their partners; in these special needs populations this may not always be possible. Nevertheless, within society and within specific subsections of the community, there may also be specific cultural concerns which, when undertaking partner notification, should also be given consideration. Recognizing these concerns within the subsections of society will help to provide a higher standard of care and more effective partner notification outcomes.

The following populations might be considered as communities with special needs:

- people living with HIV/AIDS;
- men who have sex with men;
- women;
- injecting drug users;
- ethnic minorities;
- sex workers and their clients;
- prisoners;
- homeless people;
- children.

People with HIV/AIDS

Contacting this group of people may prove challenging as they may already feel stigmatized and marginalized by society in general, and often by health care professionals. There are serious implications for employment, travel and insurance. It may be difficult to trace contacts who are anonymous or multiple.

Men who have sex with men

Men who fall into this group may not identify themselves as homosexual; this group includes men who classify themselves as bisexual. Accessing this group brings with it specific problems as often their homosexual activity is covert, they can fear disclosure, blame, issues surrounding fidelity and their responsibility to their families.

Women

Often, women are asymptomatic concerning STIs and may consider themselves low risk concerning HIV. Their STI can affect their children. Many issues arise with this group and they can include concerns regarding:

- confidentiality;
- pregnancy issues;
- breastfeeding;
- social isolation.

Particular concerns may arise with women who have sex with other women they may need help from the health care worker with deciding on how to contact their female partners.

Injecting drug users

Issues of prosecution are often related to people who are injecting drug users; they are often disadvantaged because of the outcome and results of their drug use. The culture among this group might be that informing about others is unacceptable. There are problems associated with:

- access to services;
- attitudes of society and in some instances health care professionals;
- transient social networks;
- contact details such as addresses and names.

Sex workers and their clients

Among sex workers there is a strict code of practice, in so far as they do not and will not disclose the identity of their clients if they are known to them. Often the only way of contacting the sex worker may be through their place of work and this can carry risks; the health care worker needs to assess the risk to both him/herself and the sex worker. Other methods of contact may need to be considered such as using a mobile telephone.

Prisoners

There are difficulties of partner notification in the prison system and informing about others is unacceptable and may bring with it violent retribution. Maintenance of confidentiality is a major issue and the health care provider must think carefully about the safest way to carry out partner notification.

Homeless people

Access to the homeless may be difficult, and can be compromised by:

- low educational status;
- family support systems;
- isolation;
- lack of income;
- lack of trust in institutions such as the health care system;
- low self-esteem;
- no fixed abode.

Support and time will be needed to help the homeless person with partner notification.

Children

If any STI in a child is present then the health care worker must suspect sexual abuse. In this case the child must be referred to an expert practitioner who has the necessary skills to address the complex issues that will ensue.

Future developments in partner notification

There have been many new developments concerning partner notification over the years; however, much of this has been determined by custom and practice (Faldon, 2004b). Methods and procedures have advanced since the early days of partner notification, and each time an endeavour has been made to ensure the rights of individuals these have been upheld and respected. What must continue are the efforts to ensure that policies and procedures are refined in ways that reflect contemporary society while still retaining a responsive and confidential service.

According to Faldon (2004b), further developments are needed centring on, but not exclusive to, the following areas:

- intervention efficacy;
- factors hindering partner notification;
- large-scale randomized control trials to measure the effect and possibility of alternative strategies;
- accessing and addressing the specific needs of certain groups, e.g. teenagers and commercial sex workers;
- more robust and rigorous health intervention approaches;
- a triangulated approach to gathering and analysing data and trends associated with STIs and partner notification.

While the above areas are important they cannot be dealt with in isolation or in a vacuum and a wider perspective needs to be thought about. This will include operational issues such as the use of contact slips, the use of the Internet to contact partners and how the multi-disciplinary team communicates – aiming for a 'seamless' service. Physical and material resources also need to be considered.

Hence, it can be demonstrated that while the work concerning partner notification is undertaken with vigour there are areas that would benefit from closer scrutiny. It is hoped that as a firmer evidence base emerges the services offered to patients and their contacts will continue to improve.

Conclusion

Breaking the chain of transmission is central to STI control; further transmission and re-infection can be prevented by referral of sexual partners for diagnosis and treatment, coupled with education and sexual health promotion.

All those who work with people with STIs have a responsibility for the health and well-being of the patient and the sexual partner(s) of that person. There are complex issues that need to be addressed and these will include the patient's right to care and confidentiality, the law, community/cultural sensitivities and the overall public health. Partner notification interviews require the health care worker to use a variety of techniques to encourage the patient (the index person) to inform their sexual partner(s) (contact(s)) of their STI. This can be done in several ways, e.g. patient referral or provider referral; often more than one strategy may be used to identify different contacts of the same patient, for example a patient may feel s/he is in a better position to inform a main partner, but might prefer the health care worker to inform other partners. Partner notification should be a voluntary process and the patient should never be coerced into making any decisions.

There are several terms used when discussing the need to notify partner(s) of people with STIs. Contact tracing and partner notification are terms that are often used synonymously. It was noted that partner notification/contact tracing can be extended beyond the field of STIs and can be used, for example, when notifying contacts of patients with tuberculosis. The process of notifying partners has been outlined and there are several options available; working with the patient (the index case) will help determine the best and most appropriate approach to be used.

The health care worker must have a thorough understanding of STIs and the various modes of transmission and treatment options available, as they need to advise and support both the patient and his/her partner(s). Effective communication and interpersonal skills are needed to make the encounter non-threatening, non-confrontational and non-discriminatory.

Much development has occurred since partner notification was first used in the 1940s. There is room, however, for further development and a sound evidence base is needed in order to assess and evaluate the effectiveness of the various strategies used, and those that may be used, e.g. partner notification via the Internet.

Appendix 5.1

The following two examples, taken from the Australasian Contact Tracing Manual (Australasian Society of HIV Medicine, 2002), describe two types of contact tracing letter – one simple and one detailed. The samples can be used by practitioners and amended to meet the needs of the individual patient and the practitioner's organization.

Basic contact tracing letter

Date: ....

The bearer is a contact of patient no.: ....

Suffering from: ....

and was treated with: ....

....

Name and signature of health care professional [*normally the health advisor*]: ....

Detailed contact tracing letter

Date: ....

Dear Colleague,

The bearer of this letter is a contact of patient no.:....................................
who has been diagnosed with: ....

May we suggest that you make an assessment for other sexually transmitted infections, including urethral and/or rectal and/or pharyngeal swabs for gonorrhoea, genital and/or urine tests for *Chlamydia trachomatis*, other swabs as appropriate, and serology for syphilis, HIV and hepatitis B as indicated?

Our standard protocol for this condition is:..

....

For this condition treatment of the sexual partner is/is not recommended irrespective of the results of the tests.

Abstinence from sexual intercourse is recommended until both partners have finished treatment. Condoms should be recommended with all new partners.

If you have any queries please don't hesitate to contact me.

Thank you

CHAPTER SIX

Legal, ethical and professional issues

Introduction

Several ethical, legal and professional issues need to be considered by the nurse when working with patients in any setting. There are few areas of health care that are untouched by the law and involvement with the legal process may occur during the course of a health care worker's career (Wall and Payne-James, 2004).

There are specific issues that need to be given consideration when working with people with STIs. The nurse must work within the confines of the law, the requirements of the employer and the demands made by the NMC in the form of the Code of Professional Conduct (NMC, 2004a) (Appendix 6.1 reproduces the Code of Professional Conduct: Standards for Conduct, Performance and Ethics). Within this legal/ethical framework conflict can occur; understanding of the legal and ethical burden placed on the nurse may assist him/her in coming to terms with the potential incompatibility.

In an attempt to facilitate an understanding of legal and ethical issues this chapter will focus on some of the ethico-legal implications the nurse may face when providing care for the patient with an STI. In this chapter the law as applied to England and Wales is the main thrust of the legal debate, the legal systems in Scotland and Northern Ireland have their own traditions and although different from the English and Welsh arrangements there are various comparisons. The legal system is outlined and the complex issue of ethics as applied to care is discussed.

The Sexual Offences Act 2003 is considered and the new offences arising from a major overhaul of laws dating back over a century are discussed. Ways of thinking about ethics, ethical reasoning and ethical principles are also addressed in this chapter.

The law

Orderly behaviour in a collective society is governed by rules, and these rules are referred to in this context as laws. Wall and Payne-James (2004) state that this law is an official expression of the formal institutionalization of the enforcement of these rules through:

* promulgation
* adjudication
* enforcement.

To understand how the three points above are operated, they need to be organized and a system is required to do this; this occurs through the courts. The principal source of law is Parliament.

Sources of law

There are two primary forms of law that emanate through statute and common law:

* Statute or primary legislation is established through Acts of Parliament. Law-making abilities are given to Parliament by society as it is society that elects the Parliament. There are various stages proposed and legislative law must pass through prior to its becoming enforceable. An Act of Parliament does not become statute until it has passed through both Houses of Parliament (the House of Commons and the House of Lords) and receives Royal Assent. Secondary legislation is the making of regulations by statutory instruments. Wall and Payne-James (2004) estimate that there are over 3000 statutory instruments produced each year compared with the production of approximately 50 statutes passed each year. The details of secondary legislation are approved by Parliament and prepared by ministers; statutory instruments provide general points, and can be seen to be 'workable documents'. Regulations are often made up of specific duties, standards and procedures.
* Common law, also known as case law or judge-made law, is a law that is decided through the court system. This type of law comes into play when the courts cannot turn to a relevant statute; this may be because a particular Act of Parliament concerning the specific area of law under deliberation has not been made. In case law the courts look to precedent, considering previous cases to determine how a decision had been made and how statute has been interpreted.

The legal system is divided into:

* civil law
* criminal law

and a hierarchical court system exists where different courts administer the two types of law (see Table 6.1).

Table 6.1 The civil and criminal courts

Civil law	Concerned with the resolution of disputes between individuals (or in some instances organizations). Remedies in these courts are usually financial
Criminal law	Associated with issues between the state and the individual – crimes against the state. The outcome of a prosecution (if the seriousness of the offence warrants a prosecution) of an individual is usually in the form of a sentence or a fine – it is punitive. The outcome of the prosecution depends on the ability to establish a standard of proof that is beyond reasonable doubt

A lower court is bound by a decision of a higher court and is obliged to apply the principles of law enshrined in a higher court. Tables 6.2 and 6.3 outline the various civil and criminal courts and their primary functions.

Table 6.2 The civil courts* and their key functions

Court	Key function
House of Lords	This is the final appellate court in the UK
Court of Appeal (Civil Division)	Will hear appeals on matters of law
High Court:	Generally, hears the more complex cases and often the cases heard here are high monetary value cases. The High Court is divided into three divisions
• Chancery Division	Specializes in matters such as company law
• Family Division	Specializes in matrimonial issues and matters associated with minors
• Queen's Bench Division	Concerned with issues of a general nature related to civil matters
County Court	Most civil cases are heard in the County Court
Magistrate Court	The lowest of the civil courts

* Those under the age of 18 years are tried at special courts – youth courts

Table 6.3 The criminal courts* and their key functions

Court	Key function
House of Lords	This is the final appellate court in the UK. Often cases heard here are associated with important points of law
Court of Appeal (Criminal Division)	This court will hear appeals on matters of law
Crown Court	This court will hear the more serious or indictable offences. In the first instance it also hears any appeals from the Magistrate Court regarding points of law, conviction, or sentences passed
Magistrate Court	The lowest of the criminal courts. The majority of minor criminal cases are heard in this court

* Those under the age of 18 years are tried at special courts – youth courts

European law

In the past the greater part of European law was concerned with free movement and economic activity; while this is still the case European law is growing in other areas. European law can impact on English law. One area where European law has impacted on health care professionals is the recognition of professionals from other member states being allowed to practise in the UK. For nurses this has come in the form of two European Directives 77/452/EEC and 77/453/EEC.

The Human Rights Act 1998

The key function of this Act is to give the courts greater powers to protect some fundamental rights; it introduces the European Convention on Human Rights into domestic law. Articles of the Act can be found in Appendix 6.2. All legislation must be compatible with the rights outlined in this Act. If incompatibility with primary legislation occurs then a declaration of incompatibility must be declared.

The Human Rights Act primarily deals with interference by a public authority (although this term is not defined) on the right to respect for private and family life. Such issues, it could be suggested, are central in some respects to STI care. The principles underpinning human rights apply to all nurses regardless of their sphere of practice and they are to:

- maintain dignity;
- promote and protect autonomy;
- practise in a non-discriminatory manner.

The nurse must ensure that any patient of any age and degree of capacity can be treated with respect. Working with patients who may have an STI can be embarrassing; nevertheless the fundamental principles of respect must be maintained, in order to protect dignity, to ease embarrassment and to act in the patient's best interests. In particular there are two articles of the Human Rights Act that are related to sexual health:

- the right to private and family life (Article 8);
- the right to non-discrimination (Article 14).

Respecting autonomy means taking the patient's wishes into consideration and, normally, following them (Peel, 2004). When working with diverse populations as nurses often do, in the sphere of sexual health the nurse must also consider the legal and ethical situation concerning young people. Young people may have their own opinions, values and beliefs and if this is the case then this should be taken into account. Some key legal issues may arise when working with young people.

Legal issues and younger people

Under s.8 of the Family Law Reform Act (1969) parental consent is not required if the young person is aged over 16 years. If that individual is of sound mind they have a statutory right to provide consent; if the young person is under 16 years of age and is deemed capable of giving consent then in certain circumstances parental consent is also not required. Wellings et al. (2001) have noted that over 25 per cent of young people are sexually active (heterosexually active) before they reach the age of sixteen.

Much care is required by the nurse when assessing the child's ability to consent and Cornock (2001) states that an assessment of competence is needed. One stipulation is that the nurse must only provide those essentials of treatment that are immediately necessary to protect the young person's welfare.

In order to determine if the young person is competent in law the Fraser Ruling is applied (sometimes referred to as Gillick competence). Fraser guidelines hold that sexual health services can be offered without parental consent providing that:

1. the young person understands the advice that is being given;
2. the young person cannot be persuaded to inform or seek support from their parents, and will not allow the worker to inform the parents that contraceptive advice is being given;
3. the young person is likely to begin or continue to have sexual intercourse without contraception;
4. the young person's physical or mental health is likely to suffer unless they receive contraceptive advice or treatment;
5. it is in the young person's best interest to receive contraceptive advice and treatment without parental consent.

In *Gillick v West Norfolk and Wisbech Area Health Authority [1985]* it states that the child has sufficient:

> Understanding and intelligence to enable full understanding for any proposed intervention.

This jurisdiction places parental rights subordinate to the rights of the young person – his/her right to make his/her own decisions. Normally, the nurse should respect the young person's right to decision-making, but every effort should have been made to involve the child's parent(s) or guardian(s). If the nurse feels, however, that it would be in the young person's best interests to disclose information to a parent, guardian or social services then prior to this occurring the young person must be informed of the nurse's intentions. The points alluded to in this case were concerned with the provision of contraception; however, these details can be related to any treatment in general.

The Sexual Offences Act 2003

Sexual crime, and the fear of sexual crime, can have a profound and damaging effect upon individuals and on the social fabric of communities. The law on sex offences is part of the criminal law and deals with the most private and intimate aspects of life – sexual relations – when these relations are non-consensual, inappropriate and wrong. What must be borne in mind, however, is that law should not unnecessarily intrude on the private lives of adults. On the other hand, the right to exercise sexual autonomy in private life is not absolute and through criminal law society has the ability to apply standards that are intended to protect the public and individuals. The nurse – in any setting – must have an understanding of the issues that arise within this Act, as there may be implications for the provision of care.

This Act received Royal Assent in November 2003 and came into force in May 2004; it applies to England and Wales only. It is a major piece of law reform and has been designed to protect the public from sexual crime, particularly those who are vulnerable to abuse, for example children and those who may have a mental disorder (Home Office, 2004). This Act is the first major overhaul of sexual offences legislation for over a hundred years and the Act aims to provide a clear, fair, just and contemporary approach to this very sensitive aspect of law (Home Office, 2000).

There are two parts to the Act:

- Part I provides a modernization of nineteenth-century offences;
- Part II is concerned with sex offences. The Sex Offenders Register is strengthened and new civil orders are introduced in order to help further offences from being committed.

Non-consensual offences and the issue of consent

The Act addresses non-consensual offences and the issue of consent. The following issues are dealt with:

- rape;
- assault by penetration;
- sexual assault;
- causing a person to engage in sexual activity without consent.

In law it is vital that the meaning of consent is clear in order for judges and juries to make decisions that are fair and just. For the first time this Act defines what is meant by consent. Within the Act s.74 states that a person consents if he or she

> agrees by choice and has the freedom and capacity to make that choice.

A list of circumstances is produced where presumptions will be made as to the complainant's consent and the defendant's reasonable belief in consent, for example, if the complainant was unconscious or asleep or under threat of immediate violence. In these circumstances if the prosecution can prove that sexual activity took place and the defendant knew that these circumstances existed, it can be reasonably presumed that the complainant did not consent and that the defendant did not reasonably believe the complainant consented to the sexual activity. The Act notes that the giving of consent is active, not passive – the person freely chooses to say 'yes'.

Rape is classified as penetration by the penis of a person's vagina, anus or mouth without their consent. Rape can be committed against men or women; however, as the definition of rape states that it can only occur if penile penetration takes place, then it is only committed by men.

The new law also states that an offence occurs if there is penetration of the anus or vagina of somebody else with any part of the body or with an object. This offence occurs if the penetration is sexual and if that person does not consent to it.

Sexual assault includes any kind of unintentional sexual touching of another person without their consent. Touching any part of a person's body – clothed or unclothed, either with your body or an object – is included as intentional sexual touching.

Protecting people with a mental disorder and protecting children

It must be remembered that those people who have a mental disorder have a right to a full life and this also includes the right to a sexual life. Some people with a mental disorder may need protection from abuse and exploitation. New categories of offences have been created in an attempt to provide added protection to people with a mental disorder:

- offences committed against those who have a profound mental disorder and lack the capacity to consent to sexual activity;
- offences where a person with a mental disorder is induced, threatened or deceived into sexual activity;
- it becomes an offence for those providing care, assistance or services to someone in connection with a mental disorder to engage in sexual activity with that person.

Children are given the greatest protection from sexual abuse and a number of offences are specifically designed to protect those children under the age of 13 years; these offences carry with them a high maximum penalty. The purpose of this is to make clear that sexual activity with anyone under 13 years of age is totally unacceptable.

The age of consent remains 16 years (in England, Wales and Scotland; in Northern Ireland this is 17 years) and sexual activity with a child under 18 years of age carries with it a penalty of five years' imprisonment. It is accepted that consensual, mutually agreed and non-exploitative sexual activity between teenagers does occur; in these cases the Crown Prosecution Service will take a variety of factors into account when deciding upon a prosecution, for example:

- the age of the parties;
- any evidence of coercion;
- any evidence of corruption.

The issue of electronic (online and offline) grooming is also addressed. This aspect of the Act deals with adults who arrange to meet a child with the intention of sexually abusing him or her either at that meeting or on another occasion.

Abuse of trust

Any person over the age of 18 years who holds a position of trust (e.g. a person looking after a child in a children's home) and involves a child under that age in sexual activity will be committing an offence.

Familial sexual offences

The age relating to familial sexual offences has been raised from 16 to 18 years, protecting 17- and 18-year-olds from familial child sexual abuse. Family relationships have been defined to take into account modern society and what the family unit might be. These familial situations consider those who live within the same household as a child as well as relationships defined by blood ties, adoption, fostering, marriage or 'common law' partnerships. It remains a criminal offence for sex to occur between adult relatives in a set of family relationships.

Sexual exploitation

The Protection of Children Act (1978) has been extended to cover indecent photographs of children aged 16 and 17 years of age; an exception to this is where a couple take and possess images of each other within the context of an enduring family relationship. The aim of this is to protect children from the circulation of photographs of them, predominantly on the Internet.

There are elements of the Act that create new offences associated with causing, inciting, or controlling of prostitution of adults for gain. Trafficking offences are extended to cover trafficking for the purpose of committing any sexual offence both with adults and child victims.

Further offences

The administration of a substance, for example 'date rape' drugs, with intent to commit a sexual offence is noted in the Act as an offence. Abduction with intent to rape becomes a sexual offence.

Further offences are also included, such as:

- sex in public places, e.g. a public lavatory;
- exposure;

- voyeurism;
- intercourse with an animal;
- sexual penetration of a corpse.

Voyeurism is a new offence that applies to watching others without their consent when they are involved in private acts.

This Act ends gender discrimination and repeals existing discriminatory laws (with the exception of rape, which must involve penile penetration); all sexual offences now apply equally to males and females of any sexual orientation: men, women and people of all sexual orientations are now equally protected.

Ethical matters

Peel (2004) suggests that biomedical ethics and human rights are derived from similar philosophical frameworks. Ethical issues impinge on all aspects of care related to sexual health and STIs: an understanding of ethics will help the nurse care for the patient, and manage their care appropriately. Every aspect of nursing intervention has the potential to impinge upon the patient's physical and psychological well-being and nurses must be constantly aware of this regardless of how fleeting their interaction with the patient may be.

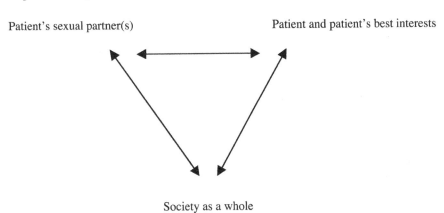

Figure 6.1 Ethical dilemmas can arise among different interested parties.

Ethical dilemmas arise when there is conflict between various interests and interested parties (see Figure 6.1). Nurses need to make decisions, prioritize care, manage resources (both human and material) and address conflict. Carrying out these tasks will inevitably involve ethical considerations; increasingly these decisions transcend technical and professional concerns (Kennedy-Schwarz, 2000).

This aspect of the chapter provides a basis for understanding ethical concerns. Key principles related to ethical theory are provided and the reader is encouraged to bring these theoretical concepts with him/her to the clinical field. The chapter does not provide the reader with the answers to the myriad of ethical dilemmas they may come across, as there are no right or wrong answers; all issues experienced are unique (for both the nurse and the patient) and are context dependent. Nevertheless, awareness of the salient concepts may enable the nurse to develop and build upon their confidence and competence.

Ways of thinking about ethics (ethical reasoning)

Nurses and other health care professionals all have the potential to affect the welfare of their patient; the ability to do this often raises issues around ethics and morals. Kirby and Slevin (2003) point out that an error in moral judgement can maim or kill every bit as much as an error in treatment or technique. Every nurse, midwife and specialist community public health nurse has and owes a duty of care and a duty of confidentiality to their patients (DoH, 2004a). Peel (2004) suggests that applying the standards of human rights will reach the same results as applying those of ethical reasoning; in health care ethics confidentiality is the cornerstone of practice. The primary purpose of the NMC is to protect the public through the Code of Professional Conduct: Standards for Conduct, Performance and Ethics; the code sets out the accepted conduct of the nurse, midwife and specialist community public health nurse. It is vital therefore that when working with patients who may have an STI the nurse is cognizant of the principles underpinning ethical care.

It could be suggested that ethics are concerned with the right versus the wrong, the good versus the bad. Ethics concern and are related to values and beliefs; ethics may be related to how we think about issues (the theory) and morals about how we act (the practice). Kirby and Slevin (2003) point out that the two terms can be, and in modern practice are, used interchangeably.

Teleology and consequentialism

Teleological ethics (or in modern-day ethics consequentialism) are concerned with consequences which may arise having made a clinical decision concerning the patient; teleology therefore could be called the 'outcome' theory of ethics. In 'pure' teleology this perspective asserts that the person making the decision must consider all possible outcomes of all of their actions prior to making a decision that may impinge on the act which will result in the best possible good as opposed to harm. Those who engage in this branch of ethics are known as 'extreme' teleologists. The key concern is whether on balance it is more appropriate or better to do one thing in terms of the outcomes the action will produce – the best balance of good over harm (Bell, 2004a).

A basic concept of teleology is the principle of utility. Utilitarianism states that an act must result in the greatest amount of good for the greatest number of people (Olson, 2004).

Bell (2004a) asserts that challenges occur when applying teleological theory to practice. The questions may arise – which consequences are desirable, for whom should they be sought and how may they be calculated reliably? The overriding principle in teleological ethics is the product of the decision – the outcome; in deontological theory key assumptions are based upon duties and principles.

Deontology

While teleology is based upon the outcome, deontology is primarily concerned with duty irrespective of consequence. According to Bell (2004a) deontology is the study or the science of moral duty. Deontology is derived from the Greek, meaning the knowledge of duty. Kirby and Slevin (2003) point out that deontologists see the acts of humans as intrinsically good or bad, right or wrong; that they act in such a way that the action is intrinsically right or wrong or good or bad.

Kant, the eighteenth-century philosopher, established the concept of the categorical imperative. This states that the person should act only if the action is universal, i.e. if everyone acted in the same way in a similar situation. This same principle also directs that person and should never be used as a means to an end.

There are certain moral principles that must be upheld when considering moral obligations. Table 6.4 provides an outline of these principles. An action is deemed right if the appropriate ethical principles have been respected.

Autonomy

Being autonomous means being in control, having a right to choose, and having the ability to act on this choice. Each person is respected as an individual when autonomy is valued. To be able to act upon choice will mean

Table 6.4 Some ethical principles

Principle	Explanation
Autonomy	Respect for an individual's rights to self-determination; respect for an individual's freedom
Non-maleficence	To do or cause no harm to others
Beneficence	To do good to others and maintain a balance between benefits and harms
Justice	Equitable distribution of potential benefits and risks
Veracity	A responsibility to tell the truth
Fidelity	A responsibility to keep promises

that the individual is rational and free to make the decision. Table 6.5 outlines ways in which the nurse can facilitate, value or encourage autonomy.

Table 6.5 Ways in which the nurse can promote and facilitate autonomy

- Choice is respected
- Be truthful; provide accurate information to enable informed choice. Information provided must be understood by the patient and given in a prompt manner
- Informed consent must be given freely and without coercion, this must be obtained prior to any action that the nurse may take (see for example the issue of partner notification)
- Risk reduction activities, e.g. safer sex initiatives can help the patient sustain positive lifestyle choices
- Confidentiality is respected and the patient is informed of any potential disclosures (e.g. when disclosing to other health care professionals)
- Patients are treated as ends in themselves; they are not a means to an end

Source: adapted from Bell, 2004a.

Non-maleficence

Causing no harm to others is acting in a non-maleficent manner. Harm can take many forms – there may be physical harm, e.g. the pain caused when taking a specimen from the patient; psychological harm, e.g. by giving a positive test result; harm can mean actual harm or risk of harm. In the process of trying to do good the nurse must prevent maleficence or remove or avoid harm (E. Slevin, 2003).

The no-harm principle can help guide the nurse to make decisions about treatment options, i.e. 'will treatment cause more harm or more good to the patient?' Prior to considering treatment Olson (2004) suggests that the following issues should be considered:

- The treatment must offer a reasonable prospect of benefit.
- It must not involve excessive expense, pain or other inconvenience.
- The patient must be fully informed about the possible side effects and consequences.

Beneficence

When acting in a beneficent manner the nurse must be committed to doing good and acting in the patient's best interest. Beneficence has two elements attached to it: first, that benefit is provided and second, that a balance is made between the benefits and any harm. The nurse must avoid paternalistic behaviour – where s/he decides what is good for the patient, the patient must be free to act without coercion or intimidation.

In Table 6.6 Bell (2004a) considers some of the issues surrounding beneficence and non-maleficence.

Table 6.6 Issues to be considered in order to respect the ethical principles of beneficence and non-maleficence

Beneficence and non-maleficence depend upon:
- Concern for the welfare of:
  - The patient
  - The contact
  - The community
  - Other health care professionals
- Respect for dignity and privacy
- Respect for autonomy
- Professional competence
- A safe environment
- Disclosure of unsafe practice
- Evidence based practice
- Adherence to agreed policies and protocols
- Effective liaison with other health care professionals
- Ability to make appropriate referrals

Justice

The key concept associated with justice is fairness – fair treatment of individuals and the fair allocation of resources (human and material); however, this must take into account any benefits and risks associated with decisions made. Care should be provided in such a manner that the patient is not prejudiced or stigmatized on any grounds (E. Slevin, 2003); all individuals should be treated as equals. According to Lacey et al. (1997), Low et al. (1997) and Hughes et al. (2000b) the provision of a just and fair sexual health service can be affected by many factors:

* age
* gender
* race
* social class
* sexual orientation.

Where there may be unequal allocation of resources the material principle of justice is the deciding principle for the allocation of these resources. This principle specifies that the resources should be allocated in such a manner:

* equally;
* according to need;
* according to individual effort;
* according to the individual's merit (ability);
* according to the individual's contribution to society.

Conflict can occur when applying the principles of beneficence and justice; for example, should resources be spent on specific groups, e.g. homosexuals? Others, for example heterosexuals, may have their needs neglected with funds and energies being directed towards a specific patient group. In this scenario justice is related to individuals and conflict occurs when the wider community is considered (Campbell et al., 1997).

In Table 6.7 a list is provided that demonstrates what is needed if justice is to be respected.

Table 6.7 Justice and issues to be considered

Equal respect for all individuals
Consideration of the balance of benefits and potential harm
Equal access for equal need
Non-discriminatory practice
Respect for all
Priority is determined on the basis of need

Source: adapted from Bell, 2004a.

Veracity

Truth telling and avoidance of lying or deceiving others are associated with the concept of veracity. The nurse must be aware that deception can occur in many forms, for example:

- intentional lying;
- non-disclosure of information;
- partial disclosure of information.

Fidelity

Gastmans (2002) considers fidelity – being faithful and keeping promises – as the ethical foundation on which the nurse–patient relationship is based. Nurses must act in the patient's best interests as cited by the NMC (2004a) and to deviate from this may be construed as professional misconduct; the nurse is the patient's advocate. An advocate can be defined as someone who speaks up for or acts on behalf of the patient. Table 6.8 demonstrates ways in which the principle of fidelity is upheld and respected.

Table 6.8 Issues to consider when acting as the patient's advocate

The nurse represents the patient's viewpoint to other members of the health care team
The nurse's own values and beliefs do not influence their ability to advocate for the patient
The patient is supported by the nurse even when his/her decision is in conflict with the nurse's preferences or choices

Confidentiality

As in any area of health care provision the maintenance and protection of any confidential information is vital, patients (and contacts) must feel that the information they provide will be treated with respect and in confidence. The issue of confidentiality is multi-faceted and the reader is encouraged to seek further clarification of the concept in order to inform their practice; this aspect of the chapter provides a concise discussion of the issue. Failure to provide confidentiality may make the patient reluctant to seek help and treatment for STIs, or assist in the process of partner notification.

Section 5 of the Nursing and Midwifery Council's Code of Professional Conduct: Standards for Conduct, Performance and Ethics (2004a) deals specifically with the complex issue of confidentiality. There is a duty on every health care professional and every employee to ensure confidentiality

Table 6.9 Exemptions to the duty of confidentiality

- Consent of the patient
- Interests of the patient
- Court orders (e.g. subpoena)
- Statutory duty to disclose:
  - Road Traffic Act
  - Prevention of Terrorism Act
  - Public Health Acts
  - Misuse of Drugs Act
- Public interest
- Police
- Data Protection Act (1998)

Source: Dimond, 2005.

of information. There are, however, exceptions to the duty of confidentiality. Dimond (2005) highlights these exceptions (see Table 6.9).

There are regulations specifically concerning STIs that ensure that any information about any STI is kept confidential. These regulations fall under the National Health Service (Venereal Diseases) Regulations 1974 Section 1 No. 29 (as amended by SI 1982, No. 288). A duty is placed on every health service body to ensure that they take all necessary steps to prevent the identification of an individual obtained by officers of the authority with respect to patients examined or treated for any STI. There are exceptions to these regulations: information can be disclosed to other health care practitioners for the purpose of treating the individual or preventing the spread of the STI.

In 1991 Directions were made imposing the same obligations, as noted in the 1974 regulations on trustees and employees of a National Health Service trust. These are now revoked in relation to England and new Directions apply which are the NHS Trusts and Primary Care Trusts (STD) Directions 2000 (DoH, 2000b) (see Appendix 6.3). These new Directions (applicable only in England) impose the same duties of confidentiality on the members and employees of both NHS trusts and primary care trusts.

Bell (2004a) summarizes and outlines the requirements when managing confidentiality (see Table 6.10).

Nurses will be faced with ethical dilemmas when attempting to maintain confidentiality and they must use their professional discretion when and if confidentiality is to be breached. What must never be forgotten is that as a registered nurse, midwife or specialist community public health nurse, you are personally and professionally accountable for your practice and you may be called to account for any decisions made.

Table 6.10 Some issues to be considered when managing patient confidentiality

- Patient confidentiality must be protected in all clinical areas, i.e. prevent the consultation from being overheard
- All patient records, paper or electronic, must be protected and the sharing of records among health care professionals must only be done with the patient's consent. Exemption to this must be done if the law requires this
- The identity of the users of the service must be protected
- Codes and standards related to the level of confidentiality offered should be openly published
- The means of contacting the patient should the need arise must be discussed in advance
- The nurse should use discretion and tact when sharing information, e.g. in the process of partner notification

Source: adapted from Bell, 2004a.

Conclusion

In the course of their work nurses will face and have to address ethical, legal and professional challenges. The nurse can be guided in making decisions by drawing on the ethical principles discussed in this chapter, by adhering to and respecting the law and abiding by the standards laid down by the NMC in the form of the Nursing and Midwifery Council's Code of Professional Conduct, Standards for Conduct, Performance and Ethics (2004). The guidance and standards discussed in this Code can help the nurse make decisions, as the content of the situation the nurse finds him/herself in may dictate the most appropriate course of action.

The legislative framework has been outlined and key aspects of legislation have been discussed. The Human Rights Act, European and English domestic law have the potential to impinge on, and in some instances inform, the way the nurse in an STI setting may practise. The Sexual Offences Act 2003 has been introduced and this Act considers the law and sex offences; it deals with the most intimate and private aspects of a citizen's life – that of sexual relations. The key aim of this Act is to protect and respect.

Finally, as a registered nurse, midwife or specialist community public health nurse, you are personally accountable for your practice. When caring for patients with an STI the nurse needs to adhere to the standards laid down by the profession and act within the realms of the law.

Appendix 6.1

The Nursing and Midwifery Council's Code of Professional Conduct: Standards of Conduct, Performance and Ethics (NMC, 2004a)

Reproduced with the kind permission of the Nursing and Midwifery Council.

Protecting the public through professional standards

As a registered nurse, midwife or specialist community public health nurse, you are personally accountable for your practice. In caring for patients and clients, you must:

- respect the patient or client as an individual
- obtain consent before you give any treatment or care
- protect confidential information
- co-operate with others in the team
- maintain your professional knowledge and competence
- be trustworthy
- act to identify and minimize risk to patients and clients.

These are the shared values of all the United Kingdom health care regulatory bodies.

1   Introduction
1.1 The purpose of The NMC Code of Professional Conduct: Standards for Conduct, Performance and Ethics is to:
- inform the professions of the standard of professional conduct required of them in the exercise of their professional accountability and practice
- inform the public, other professions and employers of the standard of professional conduct that they can expect of a registered practitioner.

1.2 As a registered nurse, midwife or specialist community public health nurse, you must:
- protect and support the health of individual patients and clients
- protect and support the health of the wider community
- act in such a way that justifies the trust and confidence the public have in you
- uphold and enhance the good reputation of the professions.

1.3 You are personally accountable for your practice. This means that you are answerable for your actions and omissions, regardless of advice or directions from another professional.

1.4 You have a duty of care to your patients and clients, who are entitled to receive safe and competent care.

1.5 You must adhere to the laws of the country in which you are practising.

2 As a registered nurse, midwife or specialist community public health nurse, you must respect the patient or client as an individual

2.1 You must recognize and respect the role of patients and clients as partners in their care and the contribution they can make to it. This involves identifying their preferences regarding care and respecting these within the limits of professional practice, existing legislation, resources and the goals of the therapeutic relationship.

2.2 You are personally accountable for ensuring that you promote and protect the interests and dignity of patients and clients, irrespective of gender, age, race, ability, sexuality, economic status, lifestyle, culture and religious or political beliefs.

2.3 You must, at all times, maintain appropriate professional boundaries in the relationships you have with patients and clients. You must ensure that all aspects of the relationship focus exclusively upon the needs of the patient or client.

2.4 You must promote the interests of patients and clients. This includes helping individuals and groups gain access to health and social care, information and support relevant to their needs.

2.5 You must report to a relevant person or authority, at the earliest possible time, any conscientious objection that may be relevant to your professional practice. You must continue to provide care to the best of your ability until alternative arrangements are implemented.

3 As a registered nurse, midwife or specialist community public health nurse, you must obtain consent before you give any treatment or care

3.1 All patients and clients have a right to receive information about their condition. You must be sensitive to their needs and respect the wishes of those who refuse or are unable to receive information about their condition. Information should be accurate, truthful and presented in such a way as to make it easily understood. You may need to seek legal or professional advice or guidance from your employer, in relation to the giving or withholding of consent.

3.2 You must respect patients' and clients' autonomy – their right to decide whether or not to undergo any health care intervention – even where a refusal may result in harm or death to themselves or a fetus, unless a court of law orders to the contrary. This right is protected in law, although in circumstances where the health of the fetus would be severely compromised by any refusal to give consent, it would be appropriate to discuss this matter fully within the team and with a supervisor of midwives, and possibly to seek external advice and guidance (see clause 4).

3.3 When obtaining valid consent, you must be sure that it is:
- given by a legally competent person
- given voluntarily
- informed.

3.4 You should presume that every patient and client is legally competent unless otherwise assessed by a suitably qualified practitioner. A patient or client who is legally competent can understand and retain treatment information and can use it to make an informed choice.

3.5 Those who are legally competent may give consent in writing, orally or by co-operation. They may also refuse consent. You must ensure that all your discussions and associated decisions relating to obtaining consent are documented in the patient's or client's health care records.

3.6 When patients or clients are no longer legally competent and have lost the capacity to consent to or refuse treatment and care, you should try to find out whether they have previously indicated preferences in an advance statement. You must respect any refusal of treatment or care given when they were legally competent, provided that the decision is clearly applicable to the present circumstances and that there is no reason to believe that they have changed their minds. When such a statement is not available, the patients' or clients' wishes, if known, should be taken into account. If these wishes are not known, the criteria for treatment must be that it is in their best interests.

3.7 The principles of obtaining consent apply equally to those people who have a mental illness. Whilst you should be involved in their assessment, it will also be necessary to involve relevant people close to them; this may include a psychiatrist. When patients and clients are detained under statutory powers (mental health acts), you must ensure that you know the circumstances and safeguards needed for providing treatment and care without consent.

3.8 In emergencies where treatment is necessary to preserve life, you may provide care without consent, if a patient or client is unable to give it, provided you can demonstrate that you are acting in their best interests.

3.9 No-one has the right to give consent on behalf of another competent adult.

In relation to obtaining consent for a child, the involvement of those with parental responsibility in the consent procedure is usually necessary, but will depend on the age and understanding of the child. If the child is under the age of 16 in England and Wales, 12 in

Scotland and 17 in Northern Ireland, you must be aware of legislation and local protocols relating to consent.

3.10 Usually the individual performing a procedure should be the person to obtain the patient's or client's consent. In certain circumstances, you may seek consent on behalf of colleagues if you have been specially trained for that specific area of practice.

3.11 You must ensure that the use of complementary or alternative therapies is safe and in the interests of patients and clients. This must be discussed with the team as part of the therapeutic process and the patient or client must consent to their use.

4   As a registered nurse, midwife or specialist community public health nurse, you must co-operate with others in the team

4.1   The team includes the patient or client, the patient's or client's family, informal carers and health and social care professionals in the National Health Service, independent and voluntary sectors.

4.2   You are expected to work co-operatively within teams and to respect the skills, expertise and contributions of your colleagues. You must treat them fairly and without discrimination.

4.3   You must communicate effectively and share your knowledge, skill and expertise with other members of the team as required for the benefit of patients and clients.

4.4   Health care records are a tool of communication within the team. You must ensure that the health care record for the patient or client is an accurate account of treatment, care planning and delivery. It should be consecutive, written with the involvement of the patient or client wherever practicable and completed as soon as possible after an event has occurred. It should provide clear evidence of the care planned, the decisions made, the care delivered and the information shared.

4.5   When working as a member of a team, you remain accountable for your professional conduct, any care you provide and any omission on your part.

4.6   You may be expected to delegate care delivery to others who are not registered nurses or midwives. Such delegation must not compromise existing care but must be directed to meeting the needs and serving the interests of patients and clients. You remain accountable for the appropriateness of the delegation, for ensuring that the person who does the work is able to do it and that adequate supervision or support is provided.

4.7   You have a duty to co-operate with internal and external investigations.

5   As a registered nurse, midwife or specialist community public health nurse, you must protect confidential information

5.1 You must treat information about patients and clients as confidential and use it only for the purposes for which it was given. As it is impractical to obtain consent every time you need to share information with others, you should ensure that patients and clients understand that some information may be made available to other members of the team involved in the delivery of care. You must guard against breaches of confidentiality by protecting information from improper disclosure at all times.

5.2 You should seek patients' and clients' wishes regarding the sharing of information with their family and others. When a patient or client is considered incapable of giving permission, you should consult relevant colleagues.

5.3 If you are required to disclose information outside the team that will have personal consequences for patients or clients, you must obtain their consent. If the patient or client withholds consent, or if consent cannot be obtained for whatever reason, disclosures may be made only where:

- they can be justified in the public interest (usually where disclosure is essential to protect the patient or client or someone else from the risk of significant harm)
- they are required by law or by order of a court.

5.4 Where there is an issue of child protection, you must act at all times in accordance with national and local policies.

6 As a registered nurse, midwife or specialist community public health nurse, you must maintain your professional knowledge and competence

6.1 You must keep your knowledge and skills up-to-date throughout your working life. In particular, you should take part regularly in learning activities that develop your competence and performance.

6.2 To practise competently, you must possess the knowledge, skills and abilities required for lawful, safe and effective practice without direct supervision. You must acknowledge the limits of your professional competence and only undertake practice and accept responsibilities for those activities in which you are competent.

6.3 If an aspect of practice is beyond your level of competence or outside your area of registration, you must obtain help and supervision from a competent practitioner until you and your employer consider that you have acquired the requisite knowledge and skill.

6.4 You have a duty to facilitate students of nursing, midwifery and specialist community public health nursing and others to develop their competence.

6.5   You have a responsibility to deliver care based on current evidence, best practice and, where applicable, validated research when it is available.

7   As a registered nurse, midwife or specialist community public health nurse, you must be trustworthy
7.1   You must behave in a way that upholds the reputation of the professions. Behaviour that compromises this reputation may call your registration into question even if it is not directly connected to your professional practice.
7.2   You must ensure that your registration status is not used in the promotion of commercial products or services, declare any financial or other interests in relevant organizations providing such goods or services and ensure that your professional judgement is not influenced by any commercial considerations.
7.3   When providing advice regarding any product or service relating to your professional role or area of practice, you must be aware of the risk that, on account of your professional title or qualification, you could be perceived by the patient or client as endorsing the product. You should fully explain the advantages and disadvantages of alternative products so that the patient or client can make an informed choice. Where you recommend a specific product, you must ensure that your advice is based on evidence and is not for your own commercial gain.
7.4   You must refuse any gift, favour or hospitality that might be interpreted, now or in the future, as an attempt to obtain preferential consideration.
7.5   You must neither ask for nor accept loans from patients, clients or their relatives and friends.

8   As a registered nurse, midwife or specialist community public health nurse, you must act to identify and minimize the risk to patients and clients
8.1   You must work with other members of the team to promote health care environments that are conducive to safe, therapeutic and ethical practice.
8.2   You must act quickly to protect patients and clients from risk if you have good reason to believe that you or a colleague, from your own or another profession, may not be fit to practise for reasons of conduct, health or competence. You should be aware of the terms of legislation that offer protection for people who raise concerns about health and safety issues.
8.3   Where you cannot remedy circumstances in the environment of care that could jeopardize standards of practice, you must report them to a senior person with sufficient authority to manage them and also, in

the case of midwifery, to the supervisor of midwives. This must be supported by a written record.

8.4 When working as a manager, you have a duty toward patients and clients, colleagues, the wider community and the organization in which you and your colleagues work. When facing professional dilemmas, your first consideration in all activities must be the interests and safety of patients and clients.

8.5 In an emergency, in or outside the work setting, you have a professional duty to provide care. The care provided would be judged against what could reasonably be expected from someone with your knowledge, skills and abilities when placed in those particular circumstances.

9 Indemnity insurance

9.1 The NMC recommends that a registered nurse, midwife or specialist community public health nurse, in advising, treating and caring for patients/clients, has professional indemnity insurance. This is in the interests of clients, patients and registrants in the event of claims of professional negligence.

9.2 Some employers accept vicarious liability for the negligent acts and/or omissions of their employees. Such cover does not normally extend to activities undertaken outside the registrant's employment. Independent practice would not normally be covered by vicarious liability, while agency work may not. It is the individual registrant's responsibility to establish their insurance status and take appropriate action.

9.3 In situations where employers do not accept vicarious liability, the NMC recommends that registrants obtain adequate professional indemnity insurance. If unable to secure professional indemnity insurance, a registrant will need to demonstrate that all their clients/patients are fully informed of this fact and the implications this might have in the event of a claim for professional negligence.

Summary

As a registered nurse, midwife, you must:

- respect the patient or client as an individual
- obtain consent before you give any treatment or care
- co-operate with others in the team
- protect confidential information
- maintain your professional knowledge and competence
- be trustworthy
- act to identify and minimize the risk to patients and clients

Appendix 6.2

Articles of The Human Rights Act 1998

Article 2:   Right to life
Article 3:   Prohibition of torture
Article 4:   Prohibition of slavery and enforced labour
Article 5:   Right to liberty
Article 6:   Right to a fair trial
Article 7:   No punishment without law
Article 8:   Respect for private and family life
Article 9:   Freedom of thought, conscience and religion
Article 10:   Freedom of expression
Article 11:   Freedom of assembly and association
Article 12:   Right to marry
Article 14:   Prohibition of discrimination

Appendix 6.3

NHS Trusts and Primary Care Trusts (STD) Directions 2000

The Secretary of State for Health in exercise of powers conferred by sections 17 and 126(3) of the National Health Service Act 1977(a) and of all other powers enabling him in that behalf, hereby makes the following Directions:

Citation, commencement and extent
1. These Directions may be cited as the NHS Trusts and Primary Care Trusts (Sexually Transmitted Diseases) Directions 2000 and shall come into force on 1st April 2000.
2. These Directions extend to England only.

Confidentiality of information
2. Every NHS trust and Primary Care Trust shall take all necessary steps to secure that any information capable of identifying an individual obtained by any of their members or employees with respect to persons examined or treated for any sexually transmitted disease shall not be disclosed except:

   (a) for the purpose of communicating that information to a medical practitioner, or to a person employed under the direction of a medical practitioner in connection with the treatment of persons suffering from such disease or the prevention of the spread thereof, and
   (b) for the purpose of such treatment or prevention.

CHAPTER SEVEN

Working with particular groups

Introduction

There are certain groups and particular circumstances that are worthy of specific discussion concerning STIs. Some groups are particularly vulnerable, for example young people, men who have sex with men and some black and minority ethnic groups. In addition those who have been raped or sexually assaulted fall into the category of 'vulnerable'.

Mainstream services must recognize these vulnerabilities and furthermore, services should be fully accessible for other vulnerable groups, for example people with disabilities. In some areas it will be appropriate to establish dedicated services to meet the needs of these specific groups. This chapter will consider the needs of the following groups:

- young people
- African communities
- gay men
- those who have been raped and sexually assaulted.

Young people, teenage pregnancy and STIs

Chapter 6 has outlined some of the legal, ethical and professional issues associated with children. The Sexual Offences Act 2003 was discussed in Chapter 6 and the application of the Fraser Ruling described. The Fraser Ruling provides health care workers with guidance when working with those aged 16 years or under; it requires that valid consent for medical examinations and treatment be given. The nurse must make any decision based on an individual assessment of the young person, his or her circumstances, taking into account the seriousness and the nature of the decision to be made, the child's mental and emotional maturity, intellect and the ability to understand the information they have been given. The DoH

(2004a) also provides best practice guidance for nurses regarding the provision of advice and treatment to young people aged under 16 on contraception, sexual and reproductive health.

Those nurses who care for and work with young people will have to keep up to date with changes in policy, practice and the legal provisions that apply (RCN, 2003c; Dimond, 2005). Issues that need to be considered will focus around sexual health, contraception and relationships.

Defining the age of a young person can range from those who are aged less than twenty-five years to those less than sixteen years (Children Act 1989). A child becomes an adult on their eighteenth birthday when they reach majority. The United Nations Convention on the Rights of the Child (United Nations 1989) Article 1 states that everyone under 18 years has all the rights in the convention. Edgecombe and O'Rourke (2002) classify young people as those aged between 12 and 25 years of age. English law dictates that a young person is a minor until they reach the age of 18 years. A young person can legally refuse or consent to medical treatment when they reach the age of 16 years.

All young people are highly diverse, they all have their own needs, abilities, beliefs, hopes and expectations, and as such should be treated as individuals. The nurse must also be cognizant of the fact that they may be working with young people who identify themselves as gay, lesbian and bisexual and provision must be made to meet their needs.

There is a considerable concern within the Department of Health regarding the rise in the numbers of STIs and the high rates of teenage pregnancy. The UK has the highest rate of STIs among young people in Western Europe (Metcalfe, 2004), as adolescents consist of 15 per cent of the population; therefore this statement needs to be given serious consideration. It must also be remembered that many young people enjoy safe, consenting sex, often as part of a steady relationship (British Medical Association, 2003).

The launch of a national information campaign promoting sexual health occurred in 2001; this campaign included the sexual health of young people. The Teenage Pregnancy Strategy is a cross-government strategy located within the Department for Education and Skills (DfES) which was set up to implement the Social Exclusion Unit's report on Teenage Pregnancy (Social Exclusion Unit, 1999). Reducing the rate of teenage pregnancies will have an impact on the incidence of STIs. The DoH (2001c) estimates that at least 10 per cent of sexually active teenagers have an STI.

Wellings et al. (2001) report that there is an increased risk of contracting an STI among the younger population, as they are more likely to have a higher number of sexual partners and have more concurrent partners. The influence of alcohol and drug use in this age group and the effects of these substances on sexual behaviour further compound the problem (Social Exclusion Unit, 1999; Cooper, 2002). Testa (1997) demonstrates that those young people who are intoxicated are more likely to engage in risky sexual activity.

The DfES (2004) suggest that those young people from certain backgrounds or those who have experienced certain significant life events are at risk of having a teenage pregnancy or becoming a teenage parent. Table 7.1 outlines the risk factors for teenage pregnancy.

Thirlby and Jarrett (2004) provide useful detailed guidance when working with young people under the age of 16 years. Some of this guidance has

Table 7.1 Risk factors associated with teenage pregnancy

Socio-demographic factors
- Low income and deprivation
- Those who fail to achieve educationally
- Those who have not experienced education
- Being unmarried
- Being in care
- Involvement in crime
- Ethnicity (e.g. high rates of pregnancy amongst African Caribbean, Bangladeshi and Pakistani populations)
- Young age at first intercourse
- History of sexual abuse
- Mental health problems
- Smoking
- Poor nutrition

Cognitive factors
- Low expectation/fatalism
- Experimental behaviour
- Cognitive immaturity
- Poor skills base
- Poor knowledge/lack of sex education
- Poor self-esteem

Family factors
- Divorced parents
- Teenage mother
- Poor parent/child communication

Cultural factors
- Cultural openness
- Peer influence
- Religious influences

Source: Social Exclusion Unit, 1999; NHS Centre for Reviews and Dissemination, 1997; Chambers et al., 2001; and Seamark and Pereira-Gray, 1997.

been reproduced in Table 7.2. This list is not exhaustive but may give the reader some idea of the ways in which service provision can meet the specific needs of young people. Devine et al. (2001) state that young people are particularly concerned about confidentiality, and in particular confidentiality provided in GP surgeries, a fact that must be borne in mind when working with this particular group of people.

Table 7.2 Some guidelines that may help the nurse provide specific services for those aged under 16 years

- Written protocols regarding the management of young people should be produced as a matter of good practice
- Young people should be made to feel welcomed into an environment that is non-threatening
- When possible provision should be made to 'fast track' young people through the services offered
- The issue of confidentiality must be discussed. An explanation may need to be given describing the instances when confidentiality may need to be breached, e.g. the child's safety and welfare. Therefore, it is important not to state that absolute confidentiality can be assured
- The young person if he/she so requests may wish to be seen with a friend – this should be respected
- The nurse will need to ensure that the young person understands the potential consequences of sexual activity and the law related to underage sex
- Any concerns regarding a young person must be made known to the nurse manager and discussions with other staff regarding concerns may be needed
- A multi-disciplinary approach is advocated and this may include for example consultation with the school nurse, health visitor and/or practice nurse
- Where possible a designated young persons service, where young people need not see other adults attending for care, should be provided

Source: adapted from Thirlby and Jarrett, 2004.

While the issue of contraception does not fall under the heading of 'sexually transmitted infections' the nurse may take the opportunity to raise this important topic with the young person when s/he is being examined and treated for any STIs. However, prior to doing this the nurse must have insight and understanding regarding the complexities surrounding contraception and reproductive health. When the nurse addresses sexual health in a holistic manner then the issues of contraception and reproduction will need to be given due consideration.

Young gay men

Young gay men have specific needs; they may find it difficult to disclose their sexuality and as a result of this they may leave seeking help and support until the STI has advanced to the acute stage. In order to encourage young gay men to seek help sooner, the sexual health services provided by nurses and other health care professionals must be user friendly. This includes how and where the services are advertised, where they are provided and at what time.

Most young people find it difficult and embarrassing to discuss issues of a sexual nature and this is also true of young men, especially when it concerns acts of a homosexual nature. Nurses should be guided by the patient regarding the pace at which the consultation is set and the language that is to be used. It is important that the nurse asks the patient to clarify any terminology he is using that may be new or confusing; it is equally important to ensure the nurse checks with the patient that he understands the language and terminology s/he is using.

While there may be physical implications of an untreated STI, there may also be psychosexual and emotional issues that will need to be addressed. Referral to counselling organizations and support groups specifically provided to address the needs of young gay men may help; most importantly the nurse should be aware of the vulnerability young gay men may feel generally, and when accessing sexual health services.

Advice about sexual health for young people

Advising young people about sexual health can include offering support and providing information for them to make an informed decision. Young people deserve to get clear and consistent support regarding sex and relationships and this includes the advice the nurse provides. To do this effectively means that the nurse will need to allocate time to this important activity; some young people have reported that they feel rushed and do not have the time to ask questions (French, 2002). The consultation or advice giving session will need to address issues such as the emotional and physical implications of sexual activity and relationships, the risk of pregnancy and STIs. There should be no coercion and a mutual agreement to undertake the consultation must have been reached.

During the consultation the nurse should talk to the young person about the benefits of telling his/her parents and if appropriate the GP. Explanations should be given that will inform the young person of other services that may be available, e.g. counselling services or other support networks. Wellings et al. (2001) highlight the fact that none of the above will diminish the importance of parents talking with their own children about sex and sexual health.

It has been demonstrated elsewhere in this text that effective communication skills are key attributes that the nurse needs to possess in order to help people with issues regarding sexual health and STIs; this is equally important when working with young people. Free et al. (2002) suggest that a non-judgemental approach be advocated in order to encourage younger people to take up services on offer. It has been reported that some young people (Kane et al., 2003) feel that health care professionals often assume (erroneously) that the young person has or possesses knowledge relating to sexual health and they underestimate the need for more information. Kane et al. (2003) noted that the information young people would value most was information that was presented in materials specifically produced and designed for them. However, it must be noted that young people's information needs differ and the nurse needs to pitch this information at the right level with the appropriate quantity (Free, 2005). Table 7.3 outlines some issues to be considered when providing or designing information for young people.

Table 7.3 Issues the nurse may consider when providing or designing information for young people

---

- Verbal information should be supplemented by written information
- Small amounts of information should be provided at any one time in order to improve retention; too much information can be overwhelming
- Some young people may benefit or prefer more technical information supported by statistical data

---

Source: Free, 2005; Kane et al., 2003.

Other sources of information

The Office for Standards in Education (Ofsted) (2002) have noted that some parents are concerned about the suitability of some information young people receive from other sources, predominantly the media. The nurse needs to be aware of these other sources so that they can evaluate the appropriateness of these materials if they are considering using them to impart information and advice.

Television, films and friends appear to be the most important source of information for boys. Learning from other boys – their peer group – may prove to be complicated. Magazines are becoming increasingly influential sources of information for both boys and girls. While many magazines will emphasize the need for safer sex, they also appear to suggest that all young people are sexually active. Problem pages in magazines are seen as a valuable source of advice and reassurance for many young people; more boys' magazines are including such advice columns in their pages.

As an alternative method of advice giving, one NHS community trust has had some success with the use of mobile outreach services for young people. Edgecombe and O'Rourke (2002) describe how this service has attracted many young men and women. The mobile service enables young people to access advice from health care professionals in a flexible, convenient, friendly and informal manner.

Consequences of STIs for young people

The complications of STIs have been outlined in Chapter 3. In young people these risks are compounded by the fact that they tend to present late for treatment (Cowan and Mindel, 1993), they have a poor knowledge base concerning STIs and their perceptions of risk are unrealistic (Mellanby et al., 1993). Evans (2004) suggests that the undesirable consequences of unsafe sex can be prevented. Nurses, if they proactively engage with young people, may be able to provide knowledge, skills and positive attitudes in order to promote and enhance sexual health. Risk factors associated with teenage pregnancy have been provided in Table 7.1; Table 7.4 outlines the risk factors associated with STIs.

Table 7.4 Risk factors associated with STIs

- Male sex
- Young age
- Early age at first intercourse
- Number of partners
- Ethnic group (high rates of STIs among African Caribbean people and low rates associated with Asians)
- Failure to use barrier methods of contraception
- Previous STIs
- Male homosexuality
- Previous attendance at a genitourinary clinic

Source: Adler, 1997; Cowan and Mindel, 1993; Evans et al., 1998; Stokes, 1997.

In one single act of unprotected sex an adolescent girl has a 1 per cent chance of acquiring HIV, 30 per cent chance of contracting genital herpes and 50 per cent chance of acquiring gonorrhoea (Social Exclusion Unit, 1999). Costs to the individual include preventable infertility, ectopic pregnancy; hospital admission for pelvic inflammatory disease and the associated psychological stress; there are also costs to society (British Medical Association, 2002).

Suspected child abuse

First and foremost the responsibility of the nurse when child abuse or potential child abuse is suspected is to the young person. Child protection issues must be considered in the overall management of the young person (Thirlby and Jarrett, 2004).

It is the duty of each NHS trust to have a named nurse or midwife and a named doctor who takes on the professional lead for all child protection matters within the trust. This requirement emerged from the need to safeguard children (DoH, 1999b).

When working with young people in the field of sexual health the nurse must be aware of the possibility of child abuse. An awareness of local policy, procedure and protocols concerning the local Area Child Protection Committee is needed, as is the need to know the name and contact details of the named professional leads within the trust.

Forcing a young person to take part in sexual activity is deemed sexual abuse, regardless of whether that person is aware of what is happening. The DoH (1999b) defines some of these sexual activities as:

• physical contact;
• rape;
• buggery;
• non-penetrative acts.

Included in this are also non-contact activities such as:

• involving the young person in looking at pornographic material;
• the production of pornographic material with that young person;
• watching sexual activities;
• encouraging young people to behave in sexually inappropriate ways.

While it is acknowledged that some children under 16 years may engage in consensual sexual activity, the following issues need to be given consideration:

• risk of contracting and transmitting an STI;
• past and continuing sexual abuse/assault;
• undiagnosed mental health problems;
• risk of or involvement in prostitution, i.e. commercial sex workers;
• vulnerability caused by living away from home, e.g. local authority accommodation;
• vulnerability associated with those young people with a physical and/or learning disability.

If a child discloses information to the nurse concerning child abuse, with the child's consent (although there may be situations where confidentiality may need to be breached) this should be discussed with senior nursing and medical colleagues. If the outcome of the deliberations leads to the performance of an examination of the child this can only be conducted by a forensic medical examiner. The reason for this is that any other practitioner conducting the examination may render the evidence obtained inadmissible in a court of law. At any stage the nurse can and should be encouraged to seek advice from the child protection team and this advice can be obtained without disclosing any details about the child to any member of the team.

The physical signs of sexual abuse in children are provided by the Royal College of Physicians (RCP) (RCP, 1997). When sexual abuse or sexual assault is suspected, or if any prepubertal young person is being screened for an STI, the examining physician must ensure that the origin and history of any exhibit that is to be presented as evidence in a court of law must have followed an unbroken chain from the source to the court – the chain of events.

Thirlby and Jarrett (2004) suggest that the following are associated with an increased risk of child abuse:

- history of physical or sexual abuse;
- partner more than three years older than the patient;
- low self-esteem;
- learning disabilities;
- history of social services care;
- communication difficulties;
- early age of first intercourse.

Being aware of the factors that may predispose a child to sexual abuse may help the nurse when making a full assessment of the situation.

In summary, there is considerable diversity in sexual experience among adolescents; there is also a great deal of concern about the increasing rates of STIs and teenage pregnancies amongst this age group. The consequences of STIs can result in preventable infertility, for example, ectopic pregnancy and psychological stress.

Nurses need to consider innovative methods of imparting information that adolescents will want to hear, retain and use. Some nurses may feel at ease talking about sexual health issues to the adolescent population; others may find it more difficult (Metcalfe, 2004); if this is the case there may be a need for training in sexual health issues (DoH, 2001c). The information needs of young people related to sexual health and teenage pregnancy should be user friendly; nurses may wish to consider the use of newer technologies in order to get information across and understood. Some of the newer technologies may include the use of the Internet, CD-ROMs, DVDs and SMS text messaging services.

If sexual abuse is considered the nurse must ensure that s/he seeks appropriate advice and support from a senior manager and/or a senior physician. The nurse needs to know who in the trust has been nominated (the named nurse or midwife and a named doctor) to take on the professional lead for all child protection matters.

African communities

In the UK, after gay men, African communities are the largest group affected by HIV; African communities are disproportionately affected by HIV. Since 1999 new diagnoses in Africans have overtaken new diagnoses in other groups (DoH, 2004c). Heterosexual transmission and vertical transmission from mother to baby are responsible for the majority of cases of HIV (De Sammy, 2004).

Despite many advances being made in the HIV field – for example, a change in policy from a selective to a universal offer of HIV testing in the antenatal period resulting in a considerable reduction in the numbers of babies being born to HIV positive women – African women have not benefited to the same extent as other groups. HIV is often diagnosed at a later stage of disease progression, thus limiting the effectiveness of drug treatments; this would suggest, therefore, that Africans have a lower uptake of antiretroviral treatments (DoH, 2004c). In an attempt to respond appropriately to the various needs of the African community, services provided have to be appropriate to the needs of that community.

Epidemiology and migration

Globally, McDonnell and Kiessenich (2000) report that women are the fastest growing group to be infected with HIV; 1134 children between the ages of 0 to 14 years with HIV were seen for care in England in 2003. The majority of these children are from African communities; a total of 4431 men and 8126 women described as 'black African' were living with HIV infection in England (DoH, 2004c). In 2001 the Census demonstrated that there were approximately 480,000 people in England who described themselves as black African. This number represents nearly 1 per cent of the population. In London this figure accounts for 8.3 per cent of the population. The African population differs from the population in general on a variety of dimensions, for example (De Sammy, 2004; DoH, 2004c):

- age;
- education and employment;
- housing tenure;

- marriage and cohabitation;
- religious beliefs.

Africans established in the UK may have arrived as a result of seeking refuge, asylum, to study, to seek employment or to be reunited with their families. With regard to migration, there has been almost a doubling of the black African population between 1991 and 2001; the numbers have risen from 212,000 to 480,000 (respectively). Thirlby and Lee (2004) suggest that those groups who are most seriously affected by HIV are people from:

- Democratic Republic of Congo
- Malawi
- Kenya
- Uganda
- Tanzania
- Zimbabwe

Accessing and providing services

Fenton et al. (2002) have demonstrated that some members of the African community have a greater need for sexual health services; despite this they are less inclined to use or access sexual health services available. Challenges face health care providers when they attempt to encourage some Africans to access services. Many Africans living in England are permanent residents or may have limited residential status and a number are affected by asylum legislation. Confusion can arise among patients and health care providers concerning access to treatment. In an attempt to address these challenges the government and the Refugee Council have published a document, *Caring for Dispersed Asylum Seekers* (DoH and the Refugee Council, 2003); section 1 of this pack addresses entitlement to health care.

If health care services are to be accessed and used by African communities and the services provided are appropriate, it is important that the nurse considers the specific needs of this group of patients: this is the first step towards effective HIV prevention. Being aware of the local and national services available may help to provide patients with up to date and accurate information.

Many Africans may have only recently migrated to the UK; within local communities there may still be traditional practices and beliefs regarding sexual attitudes and lifestyle. The DoH (2004c) suggest that some factors influencing these practices and beliefs may be related to:

- gender;
- ethnic origin (i.e. tribal groups);

- religion;
- acculturation.

There are few empirical studies that have examined sexual attitudes, beliefs and lifestyles of African communities; however, those studies undertaken have suggested that themes have begun to emerge and include (DoH, 2004c):

- preponderance of traditional attitudes towards sexual relationships and behaviours;
- religious faith plays a significant role in the lives of African communities living in England;
- a relatively high incidence of detrimental outcomes of sexual behaviour such as HIV and unwanted pregnancies;
- in some communities older respected 'aunts' have an important role in imparting information concerning sexual matters and behaviours to young girls;
- uncertainty in some communities and in sexual health services about the HIV risks related to particular traditional practices;
- twice as many men as women have reported having a new sexual partner when they have travelled home to their country of origin;
- condom use with new sexual partners is intended but is not reflected in reality;
- a significant number of reports of STIs among Africans, despite low self-perceived risks and only a third having ever knowingly had an HIV test.

Africans can face discrimination and isolation, and experience the effects of stigma on a daily basis from society as a whole and from within their own communities. HIV may further compound this. The result of this can lead to many HIV-positive Africans failing to disclose their HIV status. Failure to disclose their status can mask the need for social and emotional support as well as delaying access to medical treatment (DoH, 2004c).

In an attempt to provide effective health promotion the nurse should take every effort to prevent reinforcement of the isolation and stigma experienced by the patient. Developing rapport with local African communities can help the nurse identify and target those in need, using appropriate methods. The role of the nurse in relation to sexual health promotion is to provide the people with the means to make informed choices about the sexual behaviours they choose to engage in, not to impose moral order on them.

Health promotion materials

The materials used with this group must be culturally sensitive and the information provided has to be culturally competent. It should also be acknowledged that needs may vary across and within communities. Some of the issues that may need addressing are (DoH, 2004c):

- basic information concerning the transmission of HIV, testing and treatment;
- cultural specific practices that may pose a risk of transmitting or acquiring HIV;
- perceptions of condoms;
- polygamy;
- meanings attached to sexual behaviours;
- reproduction;
- breastfeeding;
- secrecy and taboos associated with sex and relationships;
- information relating to entitlement of treatment;
- the implications of seroconcordant and disconcordant sex;
- information needs specifically related to African men who have sex with other men, gay men and bisexual men.

Consideration will need to be given to the way in which information is imparted; the nurse may need to assess the levels of literacy within the community. There may be regional variations in languages; dialects may be spoken in different parts of the community. For those whose first language is not English the nurse needs to take into account ways of accessing these communities, bearing in mind that some communities may be from Francophone Africa. Caution should be taken with any information that is associated with intimate sexual matters presented in print form, as the community may reject attempts at providing information in such a manner.

It has been noted earlier that most young people in some communities (young girls in particular) receive much of their information concerning sexual matters and behaviours from older respected 'aunts'. This peer educational approach can provide a valuable opportunity for the nurse to liaise with these older respected members of the community and work together in imparting information that can reduce any misconceptions about sexual health.

In summary, there are some important points to consider when caring for and working with African communities with respect to sexual health care and HIV. The African community in the UK is a diverse community and this fact must be borne in mind by the nurse. The high incidence of HIV among this particular section of our society means the nurse will become increasingly likely to be involved in care, prevention and treatment activities. Therefore, the more the nurse can begin to understand some of the issues specific to this group the better quality of care he/she will be able to provide. Some of the issues discussed in this section of the chapter can be incorporated in the day-to-day activities of the nurse; other issues may need to be dealt with on a long-term basis with long-term strategic, realistic aims and objectives.

Gay men/men who have sex with men/bisexual men

Clarifying terms

It is vital that from the outset the nurse respect the term that the male chooses to use in order to identify his individual sexuality. Jones (2004) states that gay men are men who have sex with men but not all men who have sex with men are gay men; the nurse should bear this in mind when working with men and the language that s/he chooses to use.

Some men will not identify with being referred to as gay or bisexual. There may be political or other reasons why some men choose one term above another, there are men who are proud to be identified as gay as it provides a sense of a shared identity. The term could be seen as a cultural or community term as opposed to a label externally attached or imposed on them by others. It might be that there are issues related to behaviour and identity: some men may engage in sex with other men but they may not identify with gay men. They may have sex often or occasionally with men or/and women and would prefer to be identified/defined as a man who has sex with men. Bisexual men are usually defined as men who are attracted to both men and women and they may wish to identify or define himself as gay or bisexual.

Men who have sex with men and who are from an ethnic minority may not identify with gay men. There are several reasons why this might be the case and this could be associated with race and exclusion. G. Patel et al. (1999) point out that in some cultures there may not be a term or concept that is synonymous with gay. Sexual identity for some men is not so easy to compartmentalize; it can be a fluid and dynamic entity and therefore to label a person as gay, bisexual or heterosexual can be misleading and as such can misrepresent those involved.

Not wanting to be identified as gay can be the result of society's homophobic treatment of gay men. There are some men who may have internalized that homophobia themselves and as a result of the negative treatment gay men may receive they have made the decision that they do not wish to be potentially treated in the same way and therefore reject any association with gay men.

Jones (2004) refers to those men who are 'situationally' homosexual. He cites some examples of these men, as those who are not or do not identify as gay, for example, men in prison. Other men who may have female partners and who identify as a man who has sex with another man are some sex workers – not all male prostitutes are gay.

As a result of the diversity associated with identity stated above, the nurse must be sensitive to, and as far as possible aware of, the personal situation and circumstances of the individual s/he is caring for. Failure to address the needs of all parties will mean that safer sex initiatives may fall upon deaf ears; therefore it is imperative that any attempts at reducing risk-taking behaviours take into account the preferences of the man. Any health education material produced for men who have sex with men may be met with resistance from those who identify themselves as gay and vice versa.

The nurse should be aware that some men, whether they identify as a man who has sex with other men, or a man who is gay or bisexual, may be wary of disclosing the type of sexual activity they engage in. This may be because they are anxious as to how the nurse may respond to such disclosures; they may fear being judged or patronized. Summerside and Davis (2001) have noted that some gay men have felt judged by health workers regarding their sexual activity and have felt unable to discuss sexual health needs.

During a consultation the man may be disguising his involvement with another man and can refer to a relationship with a female partner, neglecting to mention a male partner. In an attempt to avoid this the nurse should always, as part of a routine, ask if the patient has or has ever had a relation with male partners (Jones, 2004).

For the purpose of ease the term gay has been adopted in the following sections.

Laws concerning gay men

The age of consent is the youngest age at which sex is legal. Homosexuality was legalized in the UK in 1967, after the Wolfenden Report was conducted (Wolfenden Report, 1957). The homosexual age of consent has been reduced since then from 21 years, directing that not more than two men were to be involved and that any sex had to take place in private. In 1994 the age of consent was further reduced to 18 years and now to 16 years of age (the same age as for sex between men and women; in Northern Ireland this is 17 years). It is illegal to have sex in public places (what is defined as a public place is subject to legal debate and interpretation).

Since February 2000 gay men have been allowed to serve in the military services; prior to this date, approximately 200 people on an annual basis (both men and women) were dismissed from the armed services for being gay. Gay weddings do not have legal status in the UK.

Risk reduction and the gay man

Unfortunately, many STIs continue to mar the healthy enjoyment of sex for many gay men, and it has now been demonstrated that having an STI can increase the risk of HIV transmission. However, a coordinated approach to prevention of STIs, including the promotion of condom use, regular sexual health check-ups and vaccination against hepatitis A and B, can minimize the impact of STIs and enhance the patient's sexual health. The nurse should aim to establish a good working relationship with the patient so that the patient feels safe and able to ask any questions he may have.

The consultation must be tailored to the individual needs of the patient and his knowledge base. For example, working with a patient who has just begun to explore his sexuality will be different from the discussion that ensues with the patient who is confident in his sexual orientation; knowing the patient therefore is crucial.

The following list has been provided by Jones (2004) who suggests that these topics are relevant when conducting an interview:

- general information related to STIs;
- safer sex activities and risk reduction;
- HIV transmission;
- hepatitis A and B vaccinations;
- hepatitis C – transmission and risks;
- any other concerns the patient may have.

Time should be spent with the patient discussing the above issues in such a way that he can understand the implications of STIs and the potential damage they may cause to his health. It is also important that the nurse does not stereotype or assume anything about the patient; for example, making the assumption that the patient engages in anal intercourse based on the fact that he is a gay man: not all gay men participate in anal sex; some do not like it or want to do it and for others they may only engage in it infrequently. Johnson et al. (1994) have suggested that about two-thirds of men who have had any sexual experience with another man in their lives have never had anal sex at all.

Providing sexual health information per se is complex; providing sexual health information for men who are HIV positive is also complicated. Issues for this particular group of men may centre on risk-taking activities and the reduction of risky behaviour. There may be concerns about condom use with regular partners, condom use with another HIV-positive man and the risks of super-infection with another strain of HIV.

The information the nurse provides may go some way to helping the patient make informed decisions about very complex issues; therefore this information must be based on the best available evidence. Information and advice that is provided should be realistic, achievable, unbiased and clear. If the nurse feels s/he is unable to provide the information required s/he must refer the patient to an appropriate agency, e.g. gay men's self-help groups (workshops) that focus upon risk-reducing behaviours and general sexual health well-being. The choices that men make regarding their sexual health should be respected, regardless of that choice.

Health promotion materials

The information and advice provided by the nurse in a verbal form can be supplemented by written material. Images used should reflect the client group – gay men – and they should portray same-sex couples regarding STIs, this includes all media, for example, posters and leaflets. One of the difficulties of producing information for gay men is that terms change over time. Materials produced need to use obvious and accessible language; this means that a mix of technical and common words describing anatomy and behaviour associated with sex will be needed.

However, there may be instances when it is inappropriate to provide gay men with written material as described above. In some instances, for example, if a man is living with others who are unaware of his sexuality, then the written material provided should be 'general' in nature, so that it will not identify him as a man who has sex with other men.

This aspect of the chapter has briefly considered the needs of gay men. Men who engage in homosexual activity use various terms to define and identify themselves, for example 'gay', 'bisexual' and 'men who have sex with men'. If the nurse is to fully engage gay men in sexual health promotion and risk-taking initiatives then s/he must respect the term used by the man to define/identify himself.

Health promotion activities must be evidence based in order to help men make informed decisions. The materials used will ideally reflect the client group and use the language that the man can relate to.

Adult survivors of acute sexual assault

Child abuse has already been discussed earlier; this aspect of the chapter will briefly consider those who have been raped and/or subjected to sexual abuse.

Survivors of sexual assault can experience a wide range of psychological and emotional disorders which can include shock, anxiety, depression, post-traumatic stress disorder and other trauma-related mental health issues. They may also experience disturbed sleep, loss of self-esteem, sexual dysfunctions and behavioural and eating disorders. Psychological and emotional trauma can also manifest itself in physical reactions such as stomach-aches, headaches and back problems. It has also been noted that sexual assault victims are more likely to attempt, or to commit suicide (WHO, 2002b).

Spitzberg (1999) has estimated that approximately 13 per cent of women and 3 per cent of men worldwide may be raped at some time during their lives. However, this data should be treated with caution as reliable incidence figures are impossible to estimate as a result of the barriers to reporting that sexual assault presents, often unexpectedly, to health care providers working in diverse areas.

The law has defined rape and sexual assault in the Sexual Offences Act 2003. It is a myth that rape and sexual assault can only be perpetrated on women by men; both men and women may experience the trauma of rape and sexual assault by the opposite or the same sex. Sexual assault occurs in every society; it constitutes a violation of basic human rights (United Nations High Commissioner for Refugees, 1995).

The nurse should aim to provide the patient with an all-inclusive sexual health service that is sensitive, compassionate, discreet and respectful.

Protocols and policies should be available to nurses, midwives and/or specialist community public health nurses who are working in specific care settings, for example (but not exclusively) genitourinary medicine and accident and emergency settings. When a multidisciplinary approach has been taken to devise policy and protocol the team must also take into account local and national policy. National guidelines have been devised by the Association for Genitourinary Medicine and the Medical Society for the Study of Venereal Diseases (AGUM and MSSVD, 2001) regarding the management of adult victims of sexual assault.

Examination and assessment

Care for the victim must only be limited to the diagnosis, treatment and psychological support; an examination required for the collection of specimens for forensic purposes must not be undertaken by the nurse. If the patient decides to undergo a forensic examination then no other examination must be performed as this may invalidate any evidence collected during the forensic examination. The approach used must be one that deals compassionately with the patient's psychological condition; the nurse as the patient's advocate has to balance the need of taking specimens against the patient's suffering.

The investigations required will be carried out according to need, e.g. STI screening, pregnancy testing and HIV assessment; these investigations will vary in accordance with local policy. Reynolds et al. (2000) note that survivors of sexual assault have higher rates of STIs compared with the general population; therefore opportunist screening may be beneficial. The following issues will need to be addressed if a patient requests an examination (Reynolds et al., 2000; Wakley et al., 2003):

- provision of emergency contraception (if appropriate);
- screening for STIs;
  - gonorrhoea;
  - chlamydia;
  - bacterial vaginosis;
  - *Trichomonas vaginalis;*
  - blood for syphilis;
  - hepatitis B and C, HIV testing (if indicated);
- provision of antibiotic therapy;
- provision of post-exposure prophylaxis (HIV) therapy (if indicated);
- provision of hepatitis B vaccination (if appropriate);
- provision of emotional and psychosexual support if needed (consider referral for counselling);
- analgesia may be required;
- tetanus toxoid (if appropriate).

Depending on the patient's contraceptive history and menstrual cycle, testing of urine or blood will dictate treatment and follow-up with respect to pregnancy risk. There is a risk of HIV transmission from one act of unprotected penetrative intercourse; however, this risk is very low. If the assault included unprotected anal or vaginal intercourse then the patient is advised to use a condom until the diagnosis of HIV has been ruled out – usually within three months (Mein et al., 2003).

The forensic examination

Rogers (1996) recommends that a physician trained in forensic medicine is required to undertake this specific activity. If the patient has reported the incident to the police then a forensic examination will have already been undertaken; the forensic examination may not have included screening for and treatment of STIs. The treatment of any injuries sustained during the assault takes priority over the examination and if the assault has occurred recently then immediate medical care may be needed. The overall aim of this examination is to gather evidence for any legal proceedings that may take place.

The patient may decline a forensic examination. The nurse will need to determine if a patient prefers a same-sex health care practitioner to undertake the examination. The nurse must be guided by the patient's best interests and respect the person's wishes in all instances.

DNA evidence left on or in the body of the survivor, in moist areas, degrades quickly; often this is over 2–10 days. Forensic examination therefore needs to be conducted as soon as possible but within 10 days of an assault (Hampton, 1995). If the patient agrees to undergo a forensic examination then they should be advised as follows:

- Do not shower or bathe.
- Do not clean the teeth or rinse the mouth out.
- Ensure all clothes worn remain unwashed.

Note: the patient should be asked to store underclothes worn during the assault in paper bags not plastic bags in order to reduce the speed at which the DNA degrades.

Sexual assault and the risk of HIV and STIs

For those survivors of sexual assault or rape they may be at increased risk of HIV and/or other STIs as a result of:

- the use of force may have been traumatic to the genital tract (tearing injury), increasing the risk of contracting HIV;
- perpetrators tend to belong to a category of individuals who have higher rates of STIs;
- a co-infection with an STI may also increase the risk of HIV transmission.

Legal support may also be needed if the patient wishes to proceed with legal charges; the nurse can act as the coordinator if referral is required. This section of the chapter has briefly considered adult acute sexual assault. The nurse can assist the survivor from a physical and psychological perspective. If the patient wishes to undergo a forensic examination then only an appropriately trained person can conduct this examination and no other examination should be conducted. If the patient decides not to proceed with a forensic examination (and this is their choice) then an examination to screen and treat any potential STIs should be carried out.

It may be appropriate to offer emergency contraception, hepatitis B vaccination and post-exposure prophylaxis after an unprotected assault. The survivor should be offered counselling and a follow-up appointment must be made to determine the effects of treatment and assess how the person is coping. Most importantly the care offered must be non-judgemental, sympathetic and discrete.

Conclusion

In this chapter the following have been discussed and described as vulnerable:

- young people;
- African communities;
- men who have sex with men;
- those who have been raped and sexually assaulted.

It should be noted that this is not an exhaustive list and many other groups of people could have been added to this list, for example people with learning disabilities, the prison population and commercial sex workers. Service providers must recognize and provide for the needs of all groups in society.

There are professional, legal and ethical issues that the nurse needs to consider when addressing the needs of young people. In particular the giving of information and the provision of treatment are complicated as they may require the consent of both the young person and/or the parents/guardians. The nurse must consider the Fraser Ruling when addressing consent, examination and treatment. Being aware of the challenges young people face when coming to terms with and understanding the complexities of sexual health may help the nurse provide a service that is appropriate and effective. The key responsibility of the nurse when caring for young people who may have been, or who are suspected of having been, a victim of sexual abuse is to that young person.

The largest group affected by HIV in the UK after gay men is the African community; heterosexual transmission is responsible for the majority of cases. The African population differs from the general population in many ways, e.g. age, religious beliefs, education and employment. Access to sexual health services by the African community is challenging and the nurse needs to devise strategies that can encourage the uptake of sexual health services by this group in society. Consideration needs to be given to the specific needs of the group, as this is the first step towards sex health promotion.

Men who have sex with men, gay men and bisexual men are a diverse group of individuals and the nurse should respect the term that the man uses in order to identify his sexuality. There are many reasons why one term may be preferred over another. A coordinated approach to the management of STIs within this group is advocated. This approach includes promoting the use of condoms, regular sexual health check-ups and the offer of vaccinations against hepatitis A and B. One sub-group within this group that needs to be given consideration is gay men who are HIV positive. The nurse may need to focus on risk-taking activities, reducing risky behaviour and the implications of seroconcordant and disconcordant sex.

Sexual abuse and rape can occur within any community and the survivors of sexual abuse require a range of psychological, physical and emotional support. A sensitive, compassionate and discreet approach to care is required for the patient. If the patient wishes, a forensic examination may be undertaken and if this is the case then no other examination must occur. A trained and skilled forensic examiner is the only person who should undertake this examination; failure to do this may result in the evidence being inadmissible in a court of law. If the patient decides (and it is his/her decision) not to undergo a forensic examination then screening for and treatment of any potential STIs will be carried out. The patient may, if deemed appropriate, be offered emergency contraception, post-exposure prophylaxis, vaccinations for hepatitis B and tetanus toxoid. The survivor may benefit from counselling in order to deal with any emotional/psychological issues that could arise as a result of the attack.

Glossary

Advocate	A person who pleads for another.
Autoeroticism	Sexual behaviour that is done by oneself such as masturbation.
Autonomy	An ethical principle that refers to the individual's right to choose for oneself and the ability to act upon that choice.
Beneficence	The ethical principle that requires the person to promote good and prevent harm.
Biomedical ethics	The application of general ethics to health care.
Bisexuality	A sexual orientation towards people of one's own gender as well as the opposite.
Contact referral	Also known as conditional referral. Index patients are encouraged to inform their partners, with the understanding that health service personnel will notify those partners who do not visit the health service within a contracted time period.
Deontology	Ethical theory that considers the intrinsic moral significance of an act itself as the criterion for determination of good.
Dyspareunia	Painful intercourse.

Emotional attachment   The human capacity to establish bonds with other human beings that are built and maintained through emotion.

Eroticism   Human capacity to experience subjective responses that elicit physical phenomena perceived as sexual desire, sexual arousal and orgasm and usually identified with sexual pleasure.

Erotophilia   A positive emotional response to sexuality.

Erotophobia   A negative emotional response to sexuality, especially guilt, shame or fear.

Ethics   The branch of philosophy that deals with the differences between right or wrong (see *Morals*).

Fetishism   Obtaining sexual excitement primarily or exclusively from an inanimate object or a particular part of the body.

Fidelity   An ethical principle referring to the keeping of promises and being faithful.

Gay   A term used to describe those (male and female) who are sexually oriented to their own gender (see *Homosexuality* and *Lesbian*).

Gender   The sum of cultural values, attitudes, roles, practices and characteristics based on sex.

Gender dysphoria   A general term for persons who have confusion or discomfort about their birth gender.

Gender identity   The degree to which each person identifies as male, female or some combination. It is the internal framework, constructed over time, which enables an individual to organize a self-concept and to perform socially in regard to his/her perceived sex and gender.

Healthism	A set of assumptions based on the belief that health is solely an individual responsibility.
Heterosexism	An automatic assumption that everyone is heterosexual.
Heterosexuality	Sexually attracted to persons of the opposite sex. The sexual orientation of the majority; numerically this is the most predominant of all sexual orientations.
Homophobia	Prejudice, discrimination and hatred towards those who are sexually oriented to their own gender.
Homosexuality	Sexual orientation to persons of the same sex (see also *Gay* and *Lesbian*).
Incidence	The rate of new occurrences of the illness or a characteristic being measured in a sample population.
Index case	The original person identified with an infection.
Insertive	The active partner in sex.
Justice	An ethical principle that deals with the concepts of fairness for each individual.
Lesbian	A female whose sexual orientation is to other females (see also *Gay* and *Homosexuality*).
Men who have sex with men (also **MSM** and **MWHSWM**)	This phrase is used by many statutory organizations and health services. It encompasses all men who have sex with other men and who would not use the terms 'gay', 'bisexual' or 'homosexual' to describe themselves.

Morals   Refers to behaviour in accordance with cus-
                              tom or tradition.

Non-maleficence   Ethical concept referring to the duty to do
                              or cause no harm to others.

Paraphilia   Any of a group of psychosexual disorders
                              characterized by sexual fantasies, feelings,
                              or activities involving a non-human object,
                              a non-consenting partner, or pain or humil-
                              iation of oneself or one's partner;
                              paraphilia is also called sexual deviation.

Patient referral   Health service personnel encourage index
                              patients to inform partners directly of their
                              possible exposure to sexually transmitted
                              infections.

Prodrome   The period prior to a viral outbreak in an
                              individual when live viruses are shed from
                              the affected areas. The person is highly
                              infectious at this time, though asympto-
                              matic.

Professional misconduct   Conduct of registered nurse, midwife or
                              specialist community public health nurse
                              that may lead to conduct and competence
                              proceedings by the Nursing and Midwifery
                              Council.

Provider referral   Third parties (usually health service per-
                              sonnel) notify partners identified by index
                              patients, without disclosing the name of the
                              patient to the partners.

Receptive   The passive partner in sex.

Safer sex   A term used to specify sexual practices and
                              sexual behaviours that reduce risk of con-
                              tracting and transmitting STIs, especially
                              HIV.

Seroconcordant	A couple where both people are HIV positive.
Serodisconcordant	A couple where one person is HIV positive and the other is HIV negative.
Sex	The sum of biological characteristics that define the spectrum of humans as females and males.
Sexual activity	A behavioural expression of one's sexuality where the erotic component of sexuality is most evident.
Sexual health	The experience of the ongoing process of physical, psychological and socio-cultural well-being related to sexuality.
Sexual identity	The overall sexual identity which includes how the individual identifies as male, female, masculine, feminine or some combination and the individual's sexual orientation.
Sexuality	A core dimension of being human which includes sex, gender, sexual and gender identity, sexual orientation, eroticism, emotional attachment/love, and reproduction.
Sexual orientation	The organization of an individual's eroticism and/or emotional attachments with reference to the sex and gender of the partner involved in sexual activity.
Sexual practice	A pattern of sexual activity that is exhibited by an individual or a community with enough consistency to be expected as a behaviour.
Source person	The person from whom the index case acquired an infection.

Subpoena   An order of the court requiring a person to appear as a witness or to bring records such as nursing documentation to court.

Teleology   Ethical theory that states that the moral value of a situation is determined by its consequences.

Transgender   This term is often used interchangeably with transsexual. It is a term used to describe those people who have undergone gender transformation or gender reassignment.

Transsexual   This term encapsulates all of those people who are living in the gender opposite to that assigned at birth; surgery may not have been undertaken as is the case with transgender people.

Transvestitism   A person who dresses and acts in a style or manner traditionally associated with the opposite sex, cross dressing.

Vaginismus   A sexual dysfunction characterized by strong, involuntary muscle spasms around the vaginal entrance, preventing the insertion of a penis.

Veracity   An ethical principle relating to truthfulness – there should be neither lies nor deception.

References

Adler MW (1997) Sexual health: a health of the nation failure. British Medical Journal 314: 1743–7.

Adler M, French P (2004) Syphilis – clinical features, diagnosis and management. In M Adler, F Cowan, P Mitchell et al. (eds), ABC of Sexually Transmitted Infections, 5th edn, ch. 12, pp. 49–55. London: BMJ Press.

Aguilera DC, Messick JM (1982) Crisis Intervention: Therapy for Psychological Emergencies. Missouri: Mosby.

AGUM and MSSVD (2001) National Guidelines for the Management of Genital Herpes. London: Association for Genitourinary Medicine and the Medical Society for the Study of Venereal Diseases.

Alder MW (2001) Development of the epidemic. In MW Adler (ed.), ABC of AIDS, 5th edn, ch. 1, pp. 1–6. London: BMJ Publishing.

Alter M (1997) Epidemiology of hepatitis B. Hepatology 26: 62S–65S.

Annon JS (1975) The Behavioural Treatment of Sexual Problems. New York: Harper & Row.

Association for Genitourinary Medicine and the Medical Society for the Study of Venereal Diseases (2001) National Guidelines on the Management of Adult Victims of Sexual Assault. London: MSSVD.

Association for Genitourinary Medicine and the Medical Society for the Study of Venereal Diseases (2002) Clinical Effectiveness Guidelines. London: MSSVD.

Association of British Insurers and the British Medical Association (2002) Medical Information and Insurance. London: BMA.

Australasian Society for HIV Medicine (2002) Australasian Contact Tracing Manual. Sydney: Commonwealth Department of Health and Ageing.

Bachmann GA, Leiblum SR, Grill J (1989) Brief sexual enquiry in gynecologic practice. Obstetrics and Gynecology 73: 425–7.

Barlow D, Philips I (1978) Gonorrhoea in women: diagnostic, clinical and laboratory aspects. Lancet 1: 761–4.

Bell G (2004a) Ethical issues in sexual health advising. In Society of Sexual Health Advisors (ed.), The Manual for Sexual Health Advisors, ch. 23, pp. 208–20. London: SSHA.

Bell G (2004b) Partner notification: interviews. In Society of Sexual Health Advisers (ed.), The Manual for Sexual Health Advisers, ch. 2, pp. 23–40. London: SSHA.

Bell G, Brady V (2000) Monetary incentives for sex workers. International Journal of STD and AIDS 11: 483–4.

Bickley LS (2002) Bates' Guide to Physical Examination and History Taking, 8th edn. Philadelphia: Lippincott.

Bickley LS, Szilagyi PG (2003) Bates' Guide to Physical Examination and History Taking. Philadelphia: Lippincott.

Black CM (1997) Current methods of laboratory diagnosis of Chlamydia trachomatis. Clinical Microbiology Review 10: 160–84.

Bonkovsky HL, Wooley JM (1999) Reduction of health related quality of life in chronic hepatitis C and improvement with interferon therapy. Hepatology 29: 264–7.

Bor R, Miller R, Goldman E (1993) Counselling the worried well in HIV disease. International Journal of Counselling 16: 47–9.

Bor R, Miller R, Latz M et al. (1998) Counselling in Health Care Settings. London: Cassell.

Brewer DD, Garrett SB (2001) Evaluation of interview techniques to enhance recall of sexual and drug injecting partners. Sexually Transmitted Diseases 28(11): 666–77.

Brewer DD, Garrett SB, Kulasingam S (1999) Forgetting as a cause of incomplete reporting of sexual and drug injecting partners. Sexually Transmitted Diseases 26: 166–76.

British Association for Counselling (1996) Code of Ethics and Practice for Counsellors. Rugby: British Association for Counselling.

British Medical Association (2002) Sexually Transmitted Infections. London: BMA.

British Medical Association (2003) Adolescent Health. London: BMA.

Brugha R, Keersmaekers K, Renton et al. (1997) Genital herpes infection: a review. International Journal of Epidemiology 26: 698–709.

Burnard P (1995) Counselling or being counsellor? Professional Nurse 10(2): 261–2.

Burnard P (1999) Counselling Skills for Health Care Professionals, 3rd edn. Cheltenham: Thorne.

Campbell A, Charlesworth M, Gilett G et al. (1997) Medical Ethics. Auckland: Oxford University Press.

Carter Y, Moss C, Weyman A (1998) Royal College of General Practitioners Handbook of Sexual Health in Primary Care. London: RCGP.

CDC AIDS Community Demonstration Projects Research Group (1999) Community-level HIV Intervention in 5 Cities: Final Outcome Data from the CDC AIDS Community Demonstration Projects. American Journal of Public Health 89: 336–45.

Centres for Disease Control and Prevention (1998) Sexually transmitted disease treatment guidelines 1998. Morbidity and Mortality Weekly Report 47: 1–111.

Chambers R, Wakley G, Chambers (2001) Tackling Teenage Pregnancy. Oxford: Radcliffe Medical Press.

Chernesky MA, Jang D, Lee H et al. (1997) Diagnosis of Chlamydia trachomatis infections in men and women by testing first-void urine by ligase chain reaction. Journal of Clinical Microbiology 32: 2682–5.

Children Act (1989) Chapter 41. London: HMSO.

Chippendale S, French L (2001a) HIV counselling and the psychosocial management of patients with HIV. In MW Adler (ed.), ABC of AIDS, 5th edn, ch. 13, pp. 82–5. London: BMJ Publishing.

Chippendale S, French L (2001b) HIV counselling and the psychosocial management of patients with HIV or AIDS. British Medical Journal 322: 1533–5.

Clark JM, Hopper L, Jesson A (1991) Communication skills: progression to counselling. Nursing Times 87(9): 41–3.

Clarke P, Charles E, Cototti DN et al. (1996) The psychological implications of human papillomavirus infection: implications for health care providers. International Journal of STD and AIDS 7: 197–200.

Collins EM (2004) Male genitalia, hernia and rectal examination. In GB Altman (ed.), Delmar's Fundamental and Advanced Nursing Skills, ch. 1. pp. 90–8. New York: Thompson.

Colquhoun D, Kellehear A (eds) (1996) Health Research in Practice: Personal Concerns and Public Issues. London: Chapman & Hall.

Colquhoun D, Goltz K, Sheehan M (eds) (1997) The Health Promoting School: Policies, Programmes and Practice in Australia. Sydney: Harcourt Brace.

Conlon CP, Snydman DR (2004) Mosby's Color Atlas and Text of Infectious Diseases. Edinburgh: Mosby.

Cooper ML (2002) Alcohol use and risky sexual behaviour among college students and youth: evaluating the evidence. Journal of Studies on Alcohol 64: 101–17.

Cornock MA (2001) Ethical and legal considerations of community nursing. In V Hyde (ed.), Community Nursing and Health Care, ch. 9. pp. 188–205. London: Arnold.

Cotch MF, Pastorek JG, Nugent RP et al. (1997) Trichomonas vaginalis associated with low birth weight and pattern delivery. Sexually Transmitted Diseases 24: 353–60.

Cowan F (2004) Genital ulcer disease. In M Adler, F Cowan, P French et al. (eds), ABC of Sexually Transmitted Infections, 5th edn, ch. 11, pp. 44–8. London: BMJ Press.

Cowan FM, Mindel A (1993) Sexually transmitted disease in children: adolescence. Genitourinary Medicine 69: 141–7.

Cowan F, French R, Johnson AM (1996) The role and effectiveness of partner notification in STD control: a review. Genitourinary Medicine 72: 247–52.

Curtis H, Hoolaghan T, Jewitt C (1995) Sexual Health Promotion in General Practice. Oxford: Radcliffe Medical Press.

Cusack L, Smith M, Byrnes T (1997) Innovations in community heath nursing: examples from practice. International Journal of Nursing Practice 3: 133–6.

Daniels R (2002) Delmar's Laboratory and Diagnostic Tests. New York: Delmar.

Dean J (1999) Examination of patients with sexual problems. In J Tomlinson (ed.), ABC of Sexual Health, ch. 5, pp. 16–18. London: British Medical Journal Books.

Department for Education and Skills (2004) Enabling Young People to Access Contraceptive and Sexual Health Information and Advice: Legal and Policy Framework for Social Workers, Residential Social Workers, Foster Carers and Other Social Care Practitioners. Nottingham: DfES.

Department of Health (1992) The Health of the Nation. London: DoH.

Department of Health (1996) Guidelines for Pre-test Discussion on HIV Testing. London: DoH.

Department of Health (1999a) Saving Lives: Our Healthier Nation. London: DoH.

Department of Health (1999b) Working Together to Safeguard Children: A Guide to Inter-agency Working Together to Safeguard and Promote the Welfare of Children. London: DoH.

Department of Health (2000a) The NHS Plan. London: DoH.

Department of Health (2000b) NHS Trusts and Primary Care Trusts (STD) Directions 2000. London: DoH.

Department of Health (2001a) Good Practice in Consent: Achieving the NHS Plan Commitment to Patient-Centred Consent Practice. London: DoH.

Department of Health (2001b) Good Practice in Consent Implementation Guide. London: DoH.

Department of Health (2001c) National Strategy for Sexual Health and HIV. London: DoH.

Department of Health (2001d) The NHS Plan. London: DoH.

Department of Health (2001e) The Sexual Health and HIV Strategy. London: DoH.

Department of Health (2001f) Treatment Choices in Psychological Therapies and Counselling: Evidence Based Clinical Guidance. London: DoH.

Department of Health (2002a) Children in Need and Blood-Borne Viruses: HIV and Hepatitis. London: DoH.

Department of Health (2002b) Getting Ahead of the Curve: A Strategy for Combating Infectious Diseases (including other aspects of health promotion). London: DoH.

Department of Health (2002c) Liberating the Talents: Helping Primary Care Trusts and Nurses Deliver the NHS Plan. London: DoH.

Department of Health (2002d) National Strategy for Sexual Health and HIV: Implementation Action Plan. London: DoH.

Department of Health (2002e) Shifting the Balance of Power: The Next Steps. London: DoH.

Department of Health (2003a) Effective Commissioning of Sexual Health and HIV Services: A Sexual Health and HIV Commissioning Toolkit for Primary Care Trusts and Local Authorities. London: DoH.

Department of Health (2003b) Effective Sexual Health Promotion: A Toolkit for Primary Care Trusts and Others Working in the Field of Promoting Good Sexual Health and HIV Prevention. London: DoH.

Department of Health (2003c) Toolkit for Producing Patient Information. London: DoH.

Department of Health (2004a) Best Practice Guidance for Doctors and other Health Professionals on the Provision of Advice and Treatment to Young People Under 16 on Contraception, Sexual and Reproductive Health. London: DoH.

Department of Health (2004b) Choosing Health: Making Healthy Choices. London: DoH.

Department of Health (2004c) HIV and AIDS in African Communities: A Framework for Better Prevention and Care. London: DoH.

Department of Health and Royal College of Nursing (2003) Freedom to Practise: Dispelling the Myths. London: DoH.

Department of Health and the Refugee Council (2003) Caring for Dispersed Asylum Seekers: A Resource Pack. London: DoH.

Department of Health, Social Services and Public Safety (2003) Sexual Health Promotion Strategy and Action Plan. Belfast: DHSSPS.

De Sammy C (2004) Promoting sexual health in black African women who have HIV. Nursing Times 100(23): 28–9.

Devine M, Fraser J, Kinn D (2001) Confidentiality – A Training Manual for all Staff Providing Sex Advice to Young People. London: Brook Advisory.

Dimond B (2005) Legal Aspects of Nursing, 4th edn. Harlow: Pearson.

Doherty L, Fenton KA, Jones J et al. (2002) Syphilis: old problem, new strategy. British Medical Journal 325: 153–6.

Edgecombe J, O'Rourke B (2002) Mobile outreach services for young people. International Journal of Medical Health 14(2): 111–15.

Edwards A, Sherrard J, Zenilman J (2001) Sexually Transmitted Infections. Oxford: Health Press.

Epstein O, Perkins GD, de Bono DP et al. (1997) Clinical Examination, 2nd edn. London: Mosby.

Estes MEZ (2002) Health Assessment and Physical Examination, 2nd edn. New York: Thompson.

Evans BA, Kell PD, Bond RA et al. (1998) Racial origin, sexual lifestyle, and genital infection among heterosexual men attending a genitourinary medicine clinic in London (1993–1994). Sexually Transmitted Infection 74: 40–4.

Evans D (2004) Behind the headlines: sexual health implications for nursing ethics and practice. Nursing Standard 14(8): 40–9.

Fagan EA, Williams R (1990) Fulminant viral hepatitis. British Medical Bulletin 46: 462–80.

Faldon C (2004a) Partner notification: an introduction. In Society of Sexual Health Advisers (ed.), The Manual for Sexual Health Advisers, ch. 1, pp. 16–22. London: SSHA.

Faldon C (2004b) Partner Notification: Further Research. In Society of Sexual Health Advisers (ed.), The Manual for Sexual Health Advisers, ch. 7, pp. 61–5. London: SSHA.

Family Planning Association (2003) Sexual Behaviour: Fact Sheet Number Six. London: FPA.

Fenton K, Chinouya M, Davidson O et al. (2002) HIV testing and high risk sexual behaviour among London's migrant African communities: a participatory research study. Sexually Transmitted Infections 78: 241–5.

FitzGerald M, Bedford C (1996) National standards for the management of gonorrhoea. International Journal of Sexually Transmitted Diseases and AIDS 7: 298–300.

Flanagan PG, Rooney PG, Davies EA et al. (1989) Evaluation of four screening tests for bacteriuria in elderly people. Lancet 1: 1117–19.

Fletcher L, Buka P (1999) A Legal Framework for Caring: An Introduction to Law and Ethics in Health Care. Basingstoke: Palgrave.

Forna F, Gulmezoglu AM (2000) Interventions for treating trichomoniasis in women. Oxford: Cochrane Database Systematic Review.

Forster D, Pannell D, Edwards M (1999) Health promotion. In M Edwards (ed.), The Informed Practice Nurse, ch. 4, pp. 100–38. London: Whurr Publishers.

Fouts AC, Kraus SJ (1980) Trichomonas vaginalis: re-evaluation of its clinical presentation and laboratory diagnosis. Journal of Infectious Diseases 141: 137–43.

Free C (2005) Advice about sexual health for young people. British Medical Journal 330: 107–8.

Free C, Dawe A, Masey S et al. (2002) Young women's accounts of the factors influencing their use and non use of emergency contraception: a depth interview study. British Medical Journal 325: 1393–6.

French J (1990) Boundaries and horizons: the role of the health educator within health promotion. Health Education Journal 49(1): 9–11.

French P (2004a) The clinical process. In M Adler, F Cowan, P French et al. (eds), ABC of Sexually Transmitted Infections, 5th edn, ch. 3, pp. 11–14. London: BMJ Books.

French P (2004b) Examination techniques and clinical sampling. In M Adler, F Cowan, P French et al. (eds), ABC of Sexually Transmitted Infections, 5th edn, ch. 4, pp. 15–16. London: BMJ Press.

French R (2002) The experience of young people with contraceptive consultations and health care workers. International Journal of Adolescent Medical Health 14: 131–8.

Freshwater D (ed.) (2002) The therapeutic use of self in nursing. In Therapeutic Nursing: Improving Patient Care through Self Awareness and Reflection, ch. 1, pp. 1–15. London: Sage.

Gastmans C (2002) A fundamental ethical approach to nursing: some proposals for ethics education. Nursing Ethics 9(4): 494–507.

General Medical Council (1995) HIV and AIDS: The Ethical Considerations. London: GMC.

Ghani A, Swinton J, Garnett G (1997) The role of sexual partnership networks in the epidemiology of gonorrhea. Sexually Transmitted Diseases 24: 45–56.

Gibson RJ, Mindel A (2001) Sexually transmitted infections. British Medical Journal 322: 1160–4.

Gillick v West Norfolk and Wisbech Area Health Authority [1985] 3 All ER 402 (HL).

Gilson R (2004) Viral hepatitis. In M Adler, F Cowan, P French et al. (eds), ABC of Sexually Transmitted Infections, 5th edn, ch. 15, pp. 62–7. London: BMJ Press.

Goldmeier D, Judd A, Schroeder K (2000) Prevalence of sexual dysfunction in new heterosexual attenders at a central London genitourinary medicine clinic. Sexually Transmitted Infections 76: 208–9.

Haley N, Maheux B, Rivard M et al. (1999) Sexual risk assessment and counselling in primary care: how involved are general practitioners and obstetrician-gynaecologists. American Journal of Public Health 89: 899–902.

Hampson G (2000) Practice Nurse Handbook, 4th edn. Oxford: Blackwell Publishing.

Hampton H (1995) Care of the woman who has been raped. New England Journal of Medicine 332: 234–7.

Handsfield HH, Stamm WE (1998) Treating chlamydial infection: compliance versus cost. Sexually Transmitted Disease 25: 12–13.

Hawkins D (2002) Seroconversion and early disease. In B Gazzard (ed.), AIDS Care Handbook, 2nd edn, pp. 33–43. London: Mediscript.

Hay PE, Thomas B, Gilchrist C et al. (1991) The value of urine samples from men with non-gonococcal urethritis for the detection of Chlamydia trachomatis. Genitourinary Medicine 67: 124–8.

Health Development Agency (2000) Participatory Approaches in Health Promotion and Health Planning: A Literature Review, Summary Bulletin. London: HDA.

Health Development Agency (2004a) HIV Prevention: A Review of Reviews Assessing the Effectiveness of Interventions to Reduce the Risk of Sexual Transmission. London: HDA.

Health Development Agency (2004b) Prevention of Sexually Transmitted Infections (STIs): A Review of Reviews into the Effectiveness of Non-Clinical Interventions. Evidence Briefing. London: HDA.

Health Protection Agency (2004) Focus on Prevention: HIV and Other Sexually Transmitted Infection on the United Kingdom in 2003. An Update: November 2003. London: HPA.

Hensleigh PA, Andrews WW, Brown Z et al. (1996) Genital herpes during pregnancy: inability to distinguish primary and recurrent infections clinically. Obstetrics and Gynecology 89: 69–73.

Home Office (2000) Setting the Boundaries: Reforming the Law on Sex Offences (Volume 1). London: Home Office.

Home Office (2004) Working Within the Sexual Offences Act 2003. London: Home Office.

Hoofnagle JH (1990) Chronic hepatitis B. New England Journal of Medicine 323: 337–9.

Hopkins S, Lyons S, Mulcahy F et al. (2001) The great pretender returns to Dublin, Ireland. Sexually Transmitted Infection 77: 316–18.

Horner PJ, Crowley T, Leece J et al. (1998) Chlamydia trachomatis detection and the menstrual cycle. Lancet 351: 341–2.

Horner PJ, Thomas B, Gilroy CB et al. (2000) The role of Mycoplasma genitalium and Ureaplasma urealyticum in acute and chronic non-gonococcal urethritis. Dermatological Clinics 16(4): 727–33.

Hough M (2003) Counselling Skills and Theory. London: Hodder & Stoughton.

House of Commons Health Committee (2003) Sexual Health: Third Report of Session 2002–03. Volume 1. London: Stationery Office.

Hughes G, Andrews N, Catchpole M et al. (2000a) Investigation of the increased incidence of gonorrhoea diagnosed in genitourinary medicine clinics in England, 1994–1996. Sexually Transmitted Infection 76: 18–24.

Hughes G, Brady AR, Catchpole M et al. (2000b) Comparison of risk factors for sexually transmitted infections: results from a study of attenders at three genito-urinary medicine clinics in England. Sexually Transmitted Infections 76: 262–7.

International Agency for Research on Cancer (1996) Monographs on the Evaluation of Carcinogenic Risk to Humans: Human Papillomaviruses. Lyon: IARC.

Jarrett S (2004) Working with the 'worried well'. In Society of Sexual Health Advisors (eds), The Manual for Sexual Health Advisors, ch. 16, pp. 144–7. London: SSHA.

Johns DR, Tierney M, Felsenstein D (1987) Alteration in the natural history of syphilis by concurrent infection with the Human Immunodeficiency Virus. New England Journal of Medicine 316: 1569–72.

Johnson AM, Wadsworth J, Wellings K et al. (1994) Sexual Attitudes and Lifestyles. Oxford: Blackwell Scientific Press.

Johnson AM, Mercer CH, Erens B et al. (2002) Sexual behaviour in Britain: partnerships, practices and HIV risk behaviours. Lancet 358: 1835–42.

Jones, M (2004) Working With Gay Men. In Society of Sexual Health Advisors (eds), The Manual for Sexual Advisors, ch. 34, pp. 326–38. London: SSHA.

Kane R, Macdowall W, Wellings K (2003) Providing information for young people in sexual health clinics: getting it right. Journal of Family Planning and Reproductive Health Care 29: 141–5.

Kennedy Report into the Bristol Royal Infirmary (2001) Learning From Bristol: The Report of the Public Inquiry into Children's Heart Surgery at the Bristol Royal Infirmary 1984–1995. Her Majesty's Stationery Office. Command 5207.

Kennedy-Schwarz J (2000) The 'ethics' of instinct. American Journal of Nursing 100(4): 71–3.

Kent CK, Wolf W, Nieri G et al. (2003) Internet use and early syphilis infection among men who have sex with men – San Francisco, California, 1999–2003. Morbidity and Mortality Weekly Report 52(50): 1229–32.

Kirby C, Slevin O (2003) Ethical knowing: the moral ground of nursing practice. In L Basford, O Slevin (eds), Theory and Practice of Nursing: An Integrated Approach to Caring Practice, 2nd edn, ch. 13, pp. 209–54. Cheltenham: Nelson Thornes.

Klausner JD, Wolf W, Fischer-Ponce L et al. (2000) Tracing a syphilis outbreak through cyberspace. Journal of American Medical Association 284: 447–9.

Lacey CJN, Merrick DW, Bensley DC et al. (1997) Analysis of the Sociodemography of Gonorrhoea in Leeds 1989–1993. British Medical Journal 314: 1715–18.

Leach G (2004) Counselling. In Society of Sexual Health Advisors (eds), The Manual for Sexual Health Advisors, ch. 13, pp. 104–24. London: SSHA.

Lewis DA, Bond M, Butt KD et al. (1999) A one year survey of gonococcal infection seen in the Genitourinary Medicine Department of a London District Teaching Hospital. International Journal of Sexually Transmitted Diseases and AIDS 10: 588–94.

Leyshon S, Tofts D (2004) A career pathway for new practice nurses. Practice Nursing 15(8): 396–400.

Lindon J, Lindon L (2000) Mastering Counselling Skills. London: Macmillan.

Low N, Daker-White G, Barlow D et al. (1997) Gonorrhoea in inner city London: results of a cross sectional study. British Medical Journal 314: 1719–23.

Low N, Connell P, McKevitt C et al. (2003) 'You Can't Tell by Looking': pilot study of a community-based intervention to detect asymptomatic sexually transmitted infections. International Journal of STD and AIDS 14: 830–4.

McAndrew S (2000) The process: acute care. In H Wilson, S McAndrew (eds), Sexual Health: Foundations for Practice, ch. 12, pp. 219–30. London: Baillière Tindall.

McDonnell M, Kiessenich CR (2000) HIV/AIDS and women. Primary Care 4(1): 66–73.

McFarlene M, Bull SS, Rietmeijer CA (2000) The Internet as newly emerging risk environment for sexually transmitted diseases, including HIV/AIDS. Journal of American Medical Association 284: 443–6.

McIntyre N (1990) Clinical presentation of acute viral hepatitis. British Medical Bulletin 46: 533–47.

Macke BA, Maher JE (1999) Partner notification in the United States: an evidence based review. American Journal of Preventative Medicine 17(3): 230–42.

Maslow A (1954) Motivation and Personality. New York: Harper & Row.

Mathews C, Coetzee N, Zwarenstein M et al. (2003) Strategies for partner notification for sexually transmitted diseases. The Cochrane Library. Issue 4 Cochrane Database Systematic Review. CD002843.

Matthews P (1998) Sexual history taking primary care. In Y Carter, C Moss, A Weyman (eds), Royal College of General Practitioners Handbook of Sexual Health in Primary Care, ch. 2, pp. 17–50. London: Royal College of General Practitioners and Family Planning Association.

Matthews P, Fletcher J (2001) Sexually transmitted infection in primary care: a need for education. British Journal of General Practice 51: 52–6.

Maurice WL, Bowman BMA (1999) Sexual Medicine in Primary Care. St Louis: Mosby.

Medhat A, el-Sharkawy MM, Shaaban MM et al. (1993) Acute viral hepatitis in pregnancy. International Journal of Gynecology and Obstetrics 40: 25–31.

Medical Foundation for Sexual Health (2004) National Recommended Standards for Sexual Health Services: A Draft for Consultation. London: Medical Foundation for Sexual Health.

Mein JK, Palmer CM, Shand MC et al. (2003) Management of acute adult sexual assault. Medical Journal of Australia 178: 226–30.

Mellanby A, Phelps F, Tripp JH (1993) Teenagers, sex and risk taking. British Medical Journal 307: 25.

Metcalfe T (2004) Sexual health: meeting the adolescent need. Nursing Standard 18(46): 40–3.

Metters JS (1998) Chlamydia trachomatis: Summary and Conclusions of the Chief Medical Officer's Expert Advisory Group. London: DoH.

Mitchell H (2004) Vaginal discharge – causes, diagnosis and treatment. In M Adler, F Cowan, P French et al. (eds), ABC of Sexually Transmitted Infections, 5th edn, ch. 7, pp. 25–9. London: BMJ Press.

Muetzel PA (1988) Therapeutic Nursing. In Pearson A (ed.), Primary Nursing in the Burford and Oxford Nursing Development Units, ch. 3, pp. 89–116. Beckenham: Croom Helm.

Naidoo J, Wills J (1998) Practising Health Promotion: Dilemmas and Challenges. London: Baillière Tindall.

Naidoo J, Wills J. (2000) Health Promotion: Foundations for Practice, 2nd edn. London: Baillière Tindall.

National Aids Manual (2004) Living with HIV. London: NAM.

National Assembly for Wales (2000) A Strategic Framework for Promoting Sexual Health in Wales. Cardiff: The National Assembly for Wales.

National Survey of Sexual Attitudes and Lifestyles (2000) The Second National Survey of Sexual Attitudes and Lifestyles. London: NATSAL.

New South Wales Department of Health (2002) NSW Sexual Health Promotion Guidelines. Sydney: NSW Health.

NHS Centre for Reviews and Dissemination (1997) Preventing and reducing the adverse effects of teenage pregnancy. Effective Health Care 3: 1–12.

Nursing and Midwifery Council (2004a) Code of Professional Conduct: Standards for Conduct, Performance and Ethics. London: NMC.

Nursing and Midwifery Council (2004b) Guidelines for Records and Record Keeping. London: NMC.

Nusbaum MRH, Hamilton CD (2002) The proactive sexual health history. American Family Physician 66(9): 1705–12.

Nutbeam D (2000) Health literacy as a public heath goal: a challenge for contemporary health education and communication strategies into the 21st century. Health Promotion International 15: 259–67.

Nwokolo N, McOwen A, Hennerby G et al. (2002) Young people's views on the provision of sexual health services. Sexually Transmitted Infection 78: 342–5.

Office for Standards in Education (2002) Sex and Relationships. Ofsted. London: Stationery Office.

Olson TH (2004) Ethical issues. In R Daniels (ed.), Nursing Fundamentals: Caring and Clinical Decision Making, ch. 9, pp. 165–77. New York: Thompson.

Parad HJ, Parad LG (1990) Crisis Intervention: Book 2. Milwaukee: Family Service America.

Patel G, Orhan A, Maharaj K (1999) Hard to Reach, Hard to Teach: Research in to the Sexual Health Needs of South Asian Men Who Have Sex with Men. London: Naz Project.

Patel R, Trying S, Price MJ et al. (1999) Impact of suppressive antiviral therapy on the health related quality of life of patients with recurrent genital herpes infection. Sexually Transmitted Infections 75: 398–402.

Peate I (2004) HIV testing. Part 2: pre- and post-test advice. Practice Nursing 15(10): 487–92.

Peate I (2005) Examining adult male genitalia: providing a guide for the nurse. British Journal of Nursing 14(1): 36–40.

Peel M (2004) Human rights and health care professionals. In J Payne-James, P Dean, I Wall (eds), Medico-Legal Essentials in Health Care, ch. 2, pp. 11–20. London: Greenwich Medical Media.

Pellegrino D (1981) Health promotion as public policy: the need for moral groundings. Preventative Medicine 10(3): 371–8.

Peter NG, Clark LR, Jaeger JR (2004) Fitz-Hugh-Curtis syndrome: a diagnosis to consider in women with right upper quadrant pain. Cleveland Clinic Journal of Medicine 71(3): 233–9.

PHLS, DHSS, PS, Scottish ISD (D) (2000) Trends in Sexually Transmitted Diseases in the UK 1990–1999: New Episodes Seen at Genito Urinary Clinics. London: PHLS.

Pioquinto RM, Tupas EA, Kerndt PR (2004) Using the Internet for partner notification of sexually transmitted diseases – Los Angeles County, California, 2003. Morbidity and Mortality Weekly Report 53(6): 129–31.

Potterat JJ, Muth SQ, Muth JB (1985) 'Partner notification' early in the AIDS era: misconstruing contact tracers as bedroom police. Research in Social Policy 6: 1–15.

Potterat JJ, Rotheberg R, Woodhouse D et al. (1998) Gonorrhea as a social disease. Sexually Transmitted Diseases 12(1): 25.

Pratt R (2003) HIV and AIDS: A Foundation for Nursing and Healthcare Practice, 5th edn. London: Arnold.

Reynolds MW, Peipert JF, Collins B (2000) Epidemiologic issues of STDs in victims of sexual assault. Obstetrics and Gynecological Surveillance 1: 51–7.

Richens J (2004) Main presentations of sexually transmitted infections in male patients. In M Adler, F Cowan, P French et al. (eds), ABC of Sexually Transmitted Infections, 5th edn, ch. 5, pp. 17–20. London: BMJ Press.

Righarts A, Simms I, Wallace L et al. (in press) Syphilis surveillance and epidemiology in the United Kingdom. Eurosurveillance.

Roberts AR (1995) Crisis Intervention and Time Limited Cognitive Intervention. London: Sage.

Robinson AJ, Ridgway GL (1994) Sexually transmitted diseases in children: non viral. Genitourinary Medicine 70: 208–14.

Robinson KM (1998) Sexually transmitted infections. In KL McCance, SE Huether (eds), Pathophysiology: The Biologic Basis for Disease in Adults and Children, ch. 12, pp. 812–44. St Louis: Mosby.

Rogers D (1996) Physical aspects of alleged sexual assaults. Medical Science and the Law 36(2): 117–22.

Rogstad K (2003) Intimate Examinations in Genitourinary Medicine Clinics. London: Royal College of Physicians.

Ross MW, Channon-Little LD (2000) Sexual Concerns: Interviewing and History Taking for Health Care Practitioners, 2nd edn. Sydney: MacLennan & Perry.

Royal College of General Practitioners (2003) Guidelines for the Appointment of General Practitioners with Special Interests in the Delivery of Clinical Services: Sexual Health. London: RCGP.

Royal College of Nursing (2001) Sexual Health Strategy: Guidance for Nursing Staff. London: RCN.

Royal College of Nursing (2003a) Chaperoning: The Role of the Nurse and the Rights of Patients. London: RCN.

Royal College of Nursing (2003b) Sexual Health Skills: A Distance Learning Programme for the Development of Practice and Life Long Learning. London: RCN.

Royal College of Nursing (2003c) Signpost Guide for Nurses Working with Young People: Sex and Relationship Education. London: RCN.

Royal College of Nursing (2004a) Contraception and Sexual Health in Primary Care: Guidance for Nursing Staff. London: RCN.

Royal College of Nursing (2004b) Good Practice in Infection Control: Guidance for Nursing Staff. London: RCN.

Royal College of Nursing (2004c) Sexual Health Competencies: An Integrated Career and Competency Framework for Sexual and Reproductive Health Nursing. London: RCN.

Royal College of Obstetricians and Gynaecologists (2002) Gynaecological Examinations: Guidelines for Specialist Practice. London: RCOG.

Royal College of Physicians (1997) Physical Signs of Sexual Abuse in Children. London: RCP.

Royal Pharmaceutical Society of Great Britain and British Medical Association (2004) British National Formulary 48. London: Royal Pharmaceutical Society of Great Britain and British Medical Association.

Russell P (2002) Social behaviour and professional interactions. In R Hogston, PM Simpson (eds), Foundations of Nursing Practice: Making the Difference, 2nd edn, ch. 11, pp. 343–70. Basingstoke: Palgrave.

Rymark P, Forslund O, Hansson BG et al. (1993) Genital human papillomavirus infection is not a local but regional infection. Genitourinary Medicine 69: 18–22.

Sanson-Fisher R, Bowman J, Armstrong S (1992) Factors affecting non adherence with antibiotics. Diagnostic Microbiological Infectious Diseases 15: 103–9 (S).

Saurina GR, McCormack WM (1997) Trichomoniasis in pregnancy. Sexually Transmitted Diseases 24: 361–2.

Scottish Executive (2003) Enhancing Sexual Wellbeing in Scotland: A Sexual Health and Relationship Strategy: Proposal to the Scottish Executive. Edinburgh: Scottish Executive.

Scriven A (2001) Issues concerned with theory and practice. In A Scriven, J Orme (eds), Health Promotion: Professional Perspectives, 2nd edn, Part 1, pp. 7–22. Basingstoke: Palgrave.

Seamark CJ, Pereira-Gray DJ (1997) Like mother, like daughter: a general practice survey of maternal influences on teenage pregnancy. British Journal of General Practice 47(416): 175–6.

Seedhouse D (1986) Health: the Foundations for Achievement. Chichester: Wiley.

Seedhouse D (1997) Health Promotion. Philosophy, Prejudice and Practice. Chichester: Wiley.

Sexual Offences Act (2003) Elizabeth II. Chapter 42. London: Stationery Office

Sherrard J, Barlow D (1996) Gonorrhoea in men: clinical and diagnostic aspects. Genitourinary Medicine 72: 422–6.

Simms I, Fenton KA, Ashton M et al. (in press) The re-emergence of syphilis in the UK: the new epidemic phases. Sexually Transmitted Diseases.

Slevin E (2003) Empirical knowing: a knowledge base for nursing practice. In L Basford, O Slevin (eds), Theory and Practice of Nursing: An Integrated Approach to Caring Practice, 2nd edn, ch. 10, pp. 172–85. Cheltenham: Nelson Thornes.

Slevin O (2003) Therapeutic intervention in nursing. In L Basford, O Slevin (eds), Theory and Practice of Nursing, 2nd edn, ch. 30, pp. 533–68. Cheltenham: Nelson Thornes.

Social Exclusion Unit (1999) Teenage Pregnancy: A Report from the Social Exclusion Unit. London: Stationery Office.

Sonnex C, Scholefield JH, Kocjan G et al. (1991) Anal human papillomavirus infection in heterosexuals with genital warts: prevalence and relation with sexual behaviour. British Medical Journal 303: 1243.

Sorvillo F, Kerndt PR (1998) Trichomonas vaginalis and amplification of HIV – 1 transmission. Lancet 351: 213–14.

Spitzberg BH (1999) An analysis of empirical estimates of sexual aggression victimisation and perpetration. Violence and Victims 14: 241–60.

Stokes T (1997) Screening for chlamydia in general practice: a literature review and summary of the evidence. Journal of Public Health Medicine 19: 222–3.

Sully PC (2003) Communication in adult nursing. In C Brooker, M Nichol (eds), Nursing Adults: The Practice of Caring, ch. 3, pp. 39–56. Edinburgh: Mosby.

Taylor C, Lillis C, LeMone P (ed.) (2005) Fundamentals of Nursing: The Art and Science of Nursing Care, 5th edn. Philadelphia: Lippincott.

Terence Higgins Trust (2004) Blueprint for the Future: Modernising HIV and Sexual Health Services. A Policy Report. London: THT.

Testa M (1997) Alcohol and risky sexual behavior: event-based analyses among a sample of high-risk women. Psychology and Addictive Behavior 11: 190–210.

Thirlby D, Jarrett S (2004) Working with young people. In Society of Sexual Health Advisors (ed.), The Manual for Sexual Advisors, ch. 33, pp. 314–23. London: SSHA.

Thirlby D, Lee K (2004) Working with African people. In Society of Sexual Health Advisors (ed.), The Manual for Sexual Advisors, ch. 32, pp. 310–13. London: SSHA.

Tomlinson J (1998) The ABC of sexual health: taking a sexual history. British Medical Journal 317: 1573–6.

Toomey KE, Rothenberg RB (2000) Sex and cyberspace – virtual networks leading to high risk sex. Journal of the American Medical Association 284: 485–7.

United Nations (1989) The United Nations Convention on the Rights of the Child. Geneva: United Nations.

United Nations High Commissioner for Refugees (1995) Sexual Violence Against Refugees: Guidelines on Prevention and Response. Geneva: UNHCR.

Verhoeven V, Bovijn K, Helder A et al. (2003) Discussing STIs: doctors are from Mars, patients from Venus. Family Practice 20(1): 11–15.

Wakley G, Chambers R (2002) Sexual Matters in Primary Health Care. Oxford: Radcliffe Press.

Wakley G, Cunnion M, Chambers R (2003) Improving Sexual Health Advice. Oxford: Radcliffe Press.

Wall I, Payne-James J (2004) Legal institutions and the legal process. In J Payne-James, P Dean, I Wall (eds), Medico-Legal Essentials in Health Care, ch. 1, pp. 1–9. London: Greenwich Medical Media.

Wallace LA (2003) Syphilis in Scotland 2003. Scottish Centre for Infection and Environmental Health Weekly Report 38: 38–9.

Wallace LA, Young H, Codere G et al. (2004) Genital herpes simplex, genital chlamydia and gonorrhoea infection in Scotland: laboratory diagnoses 1993–2003. Scottish Centre for Infection and Environmental Health Weekly Report 39(9): 110–15.

Watkinson G (2002) Promoting health. In R Hogston, PM Simpson (eds), Foundations of Nursing Practice: Making the Difference, 2nd edn, ch. 2, pp. 26–54. Hampshire: Palgrave.

Weber JT, Johnson RE (1995) New treatments for Chalmydia trachomatis genital infection. Clinical Infectious Diseases 20: 66–71.

Wellings K, Nanchahal K, Macdowall W et al. (2001) Sexual behaviour in Britain: early heterosexual experience. Lancet 358(9296): 1845–50.

Williams IG, Weller I (2004) HIV. In M Adler, F Cowan, P French et al. (eds), ABC of Sexually Transmitted Infections, 5th edn, ch. 16, pp. 68–79. London: BMJ Press.

Wilson H, McAndrew S (2000) Sexual Health: Foundations for Practice. London: Baillière Tindall.

Wolfenden Report (1957) Report of the Committee on Homosexual Offences and Prostitution. London: HMSO. Cmnd 247.

Woodhouse DE, Potterat JJ, Muth JB et al. (1987) Street outreach for STD/HIV infection prevention in Colorado Springs. Morbidity and Mortality Weekly Report 41: 98–101.

World Health Organization (1948) Preamble to the Constitution of the World Health Organization as adopted by the International Health Conference, New York, 19–22 June, 1946; signed on 22 July 1946 by the representatives of 61 States (Official Records of the World Health Organization, No. 2 p. 100) and entered into force on 7 April 1948. Geneva: WHO.

World Health Organization (1986) Ottawa Charter for Health Promotion 1st International Conference on Health Promotion. 17–21 November. Ottawa, Ontario, Canada.

World Health Organization (2000) Promotion of Sexual Health: Recommendations for Action. Guatemala: WHO.

World Health Organization (2002a) International WHO Technical Consultation on Sexual Health. 28–31 January. Geneva: WHO.

World Health Organization (2002b) World Report on Violence and Health. Geneva: WHO.

Index